LIVING WITH KIDNEY FAILURE

Ten years ago, in the midst of a hectic life travelling the world as a TV and radio journalist, Ted Harrison experienced the first symptoms of eventual kidney failure. Four years later, between trips to Zimbabwe, Lebanon and Nicaragua, the disease really began to bite. On his birthday in 1984 his busy lifestyle came to an abrupt halt. He was given a list of forbidden foods, a regime of tablets for blood pressure, and prepared for dialysis.

Ted Harrison was still on dialysis two days a week while he was writing this book. The rest of the time he was working flat out as BBC Religious Affairs Correspondent. No way would he let the disease force him into an invalid role.

He believes that kidney patients have a right to know what is happening to them—a right to stay in charge. He believes in asking questions and making sure he gets the answers.

He writes to reassure those experiencing renal failure for the first time: this does not necessarily mean the end of an active and interesting life. He provides the hard fact information they need to make the necessary changes in habits and lifestyles.

He writes to help those in the medical profession understand their patients.

And he explores important non-medical questions: the hope and security provided by faith in the midst of weakness and confusion, and the response of different patients to serious illness.

LIVING WITH KIDNEY FAILURE

Ted Harrison

A LION PAPERBACK
Oxford · Batavia · Sydney

Copyright © 1990 Ted Harrison

Published by
Lion Publishing plc
Sandy Lane West, Oxford, England
ISBN 0 7459 1818 2
Albatross Books Pty Ltd
PO Box 320, Sutherland, NSW 2232, Australia
ISBN 0 7324 0213 1

First edition 1990

All rights reserved

British Library Cataloguing in Publication Data
Harrison, Ted
 Living with kidney failure.
 1. Kidney patients – Biographies
 I. Title
 616.6'14'00924

 ISBN 0 7459 1818 2

Printed and bound in Great Britain
by Cox & Wyman Ltd, Reading

CONTENTS

Introduction		7
1	A Series of Disasters	9
2	The End of a Lifestyle	14
3	A New Routine	29
4	Small Miracles	40
5	Moving Forward	49
6	Telling My Story	57
7	Fellow Survivors	73
8	Faith and Hope	83
9	Questions of Life and Death	91
10	Facing the Diagnosis	101
11	Eating and Drinking	108
12	A Way Forward	116
Appendix: Food Charts		123

Acknowledgments

There are a number of people I wish to thank for their help in the course of my writing this book. My consultant Michael Goggin kindly read through the relevant medical sections at an early stage, as did Marion and Geoff, Gail and Christopher, whose experiences of coping with kidney failure I drew on extensively. My thanks also go to Daphne and her colleagues at the Canterbury Renal Unit and to Cyn, Eva and Wendy at the Keycol kidney unit. I am very grateful to the renal dieticians Marianne Vennegoor, Christine Mossor and Virginia Griffith for all their help with the section on diet. And, for allowing me to reproduce previously published or broadcast material, my thanks go to *The Nursing Times* and Sister Josephine Richards, the BBC and Her Majesty's Stationery Office.

INTRODUCTION

Every case of kidney failure is different from every other. Nevertheless, by telling the story of my experience I hope I can do a number of useful things. First, I want to reassure the hundreds of people every year who experience renal failure for the first time. I want to tell them that to have a pair of malfunctioning kidneys does not necessarily mean the end of an active and interesting life.

Secondly, I hope to offer some practical advice. Developing a chronic illness does involve changing habits and lifestyles, but these changes, sensibly managed, do not need to dominate everyday life and can be absorbed into normal living without too much upheaval.

Thirdly, I hope my account will be of some value to the medical profession. Doctors, nurses, artificial kidney assistants, technicians and all those involved in the care and treatment of kidney disease need some idea of what it is like to be a patient so that, where applicable, attitudes can be examined and perhaps altered to the benefit of all concerned.

And fourthly, I hope to explore some of the important non-medical questions which arise from illness, for the benefit of the medical profession, patients and their families. The person to whom life is a great, confusing mystery can find that having a disease compounds that mystery and produces all sorts of new fears and confusions. On the other hand, a person with a strong faith can find illness a great challenge to the security offered by that faith. For everyone, illness of whatever sort confronts the sufferer and the carer with evidence of human mortality. For kidney patients on haemodialysis in particular, long sessions spent hooked up to a kidney machine give plenty of time to ponder the mysteries of life.

TED HARRISON

1

A SERIES OF DISASTERS

In 1980 I was living a somewhat unusual, some might say eccentric, life. In January that year my wife Helen and I plus our two children—David (then 10) and Caroline (then 8)—had moved from quiet rural Sussex to live in the far north of Scotland. We had bought a huge, rambling Scottish baronial pile of a house on the island of Rousay in Orkney. In order to earn the money to survive I had to commute south for stretches of two or three weeks at a time to work as a freelance radio and television journalist for the BBC. I reported for and sometimes presented the Radio 4 religious news and current affairs programme 'Sunday'. I also worked for the Radio 4 programmes 'The World at One', 'PM' and 'The World Tonight'. And, if that was not enough, I contributed regularly to the Radio Scotland news output and to various BBC Scotland television programmes.

Living on Rousay was hard work for the family but a marvellous place to return to after a hectic stint working in Glasgow, Edinburgh, London or abroad. While the winter nights were long, the summer days seemed almost endless. Sometimes we would drive in the Land Rover up the long rutted road to a lake in the centre of the island called Muckle Water, a long thin loch about a mile and a half from one end to the other, surrounded by heather moorland. While Helen and her fishing mentor, Jimmy Yorston, cast for trout, and the children amused themselves, I would get out my water-colour paints. When evening came it was still as light as day, but we would stop what we were doing, get a fire burning, put a pot of tatties on to boil and gut and cook the newly-caught fish. And just in case no one caught any of the wily, wild brown trout, we had a packet of sausages in the Land Rover.

Rousay was ruled by the weather. It was a place of fearsome winds and driving rain but also a place where storms could clear in minutes. When the clouds disappeared and the sun came out the views from the island were stunning.

There were days in the winter when the sea was so rough that the ferry could not cross and the windows in Trumland House leaked. We were lucky if we could keep a fire burning in the grate to heat just one room to anything like a reasonable temperature. Yet the sheer naked power of the elements could lift the spirits in an amazing way. There was no better way to appreciate the wonder of creation than to sit alone on a cliff top looking at the huge Atlantic rollers releasing all their pent-up force by smashing against the rocks and, over time, sculpting stone arches, blow holes and caves.

It was, as it turned out, the awesome and unpredictable power of nature which, indirectly, changed the course of our lives as a family and led to my becoming a kidney patient.

In October 1980 a devastating earthquake hit part of Algeria. Thousands of people were killed or made homeless and relief agencies from around the world went quickly into action. Within days I found myself on my way to the earthquake zone to report on the relief effort. I had been commissioned to make a radio documentary looking at the way one of the leading agencies, Christian Aid, responds to a major disaster.

A SERIES OF DISASTERS

It was the second time I had seen first hand the devastation caused by an earthquake. Four years earlier I had been in Guatemala where 20,000 people had died. I will never forget the scenes of destruction. Whole shanty towns built on rough land on the sides of ravines on the outskirts of Guatemala City had collapsed. Hundreds of families were left without homes or possessions. One day I went in a truck to the hills and saw villages, towns, hospitals and churches which had been flattened. On the return journey we discovered that the highway which we had used in the morning had been split open by a new after-shock and a long crevasse now made it impassable.

I remember one incident with some amusement. I called briefly at the British Embassy and the ambassador invited me to join him for afternoon tea. We sat in a grand drawing-room sipping tea from china cups when the plates, saucers and teapot on the table began to shake and the portraits on the wall to sway. Without batting an eyelid the ambassador observed, 'Richter Four, I would say,' and went on drinking his tea!

The sights and sounds of Algeria were similar to those I had seen in the earthquake region of Guatemala, but not so extensive. The government had taken greater control of media coverage and I had less time in the affected area and less freedom to travel around it. I did, however, have the opportunity to collect the programme material I needed to make what I hoped would be a useful documentary to raise the general awareness of people in Britain to the problems faced by relief agencies in the field.

However, reporting on disasters is not without its risks. There are the obvious physical ones. For instance, after an earthquake new tremors, often of considerable strength, can strike without warning. And there are the unseen dangers. Disasters breed disease. Water supplies become contaminated and, especially in Third-World countries, standards of food hygiene fall even lower. An experienced reporter takes sensible precautions and uses water purification tablets, but sometimes these precautions are not enough.

I think it was a plate of couscous in Algiers which did for me. I thought it had been sufficiently well cooked to kill the bugs, but from what I now know I suspect it was not.

I returned from Algeria to London to edit my tapes and write my script feeling faintly queasy. As time passed that queasiness turned into a feeling of real discomfort, and before long I had rampant diarrhoea and was vomiting so badly that I could not even swallow a sip of water without retching. I collapsed onto a bed at the BBC surgery and slept. For how long I have no idea. As far as I recall I was eventually bundled into a taxi and taken to St Pancras Hospital. Although the hospital specializes in exotic and tropical diseases, the doctors initially had little idea what was wrong with me and exactly which bug had got into and upset my system. As a result I was put into an isolation room. Visitors had to wear gowns and masks to see me and it was there that my producer John Newbury and a sound engineer recorded my programme. I sat up in bed with a handwritten script and kept a collection of towels over my head for maximum sound insulation. We could only record in short bursts, partly because I was feeling very weak, but mostly because of the noise of the ambulances and other traffic coming and going beneath the window. When the programme was transmitted on Radio 4 that evening we gratefully acknowledged the help and co-operation of the nursing staff at St Pancras.

After a few days it was decided that I did not have a dangerous infection and visitors no longer needed to protect themselves from my germs. Medically, however, I was not given the all clear. Symptoms had developed which were to hint at my eventual kidney failure. I started to produce a 'pee rose' and this blood in my urine, or haematuria, alerted the doctors to call in a renal specialist.

When he turned up he was a consultant from the old school. As far as I remember he appeared in a formal three-piece suit accompanied by the usual hospital acolytes. His bedside manner was so forbidding that I am sure he could have made a case of ingrowing toenails sound terminal. He was not a man to whom I wished to entrust my future. I was thus presented with my first major decision as a patient. Here was a man, an 'expert', who wanted to carry out tests. The very word sounded ominous. He wanted to stick things into me and grope around in my tubes and bladder to check for internal bleeding. I knew I did not want to step onto the long-term medical treadmill. I did not want to be taken in hand by the medical profession and I certainly had no intention of submitting meekly to their curiosity. I needed a plan and, fortunately, by that time I was feeling strong enough to devise one and put it into operation.

I commandeered the patients' pay-phone and called my friend Martin Claridge. Martin is a urologist. I told him my story and asked him for his advice. He said he had a meeting of urologists in London the next day and would visit me. This he did. Although he could only give me an informal opinion as a friend, his verdict encouraged me. He did not think that I needed to undergo extensive tests there and then but thought that I should see a renal physician for some checks. He would recommend me to one of his colleagues in Canterbury, Dr Michael Goggin.

2
THE END OF A LIFESTYLE

It is not easy to bring to mind all the details of the last ten years especially when, until end-stage renal failure began to approach with great speed in 1984, I did my best to pretend to myself that I was not really ill and had little to worry about for many years.

I met Dr Michael Goggin in Canterbury shortly after my discharge from St Pancras. I immediately found him more approachable than the consultant I had briefly encountered in London. For a start the surroundings were far less intimidating. I was not in bed, but fully clothed and able to enter his office as I might any other office. He offered me a seat. We talked; he took my blood pressure and generally chatted about what tests might be required. I was not at the time feeling ill and I felt, if anything, a bit of a fraud to be consulting a doctor when I was fighting fit and had got rid of all my symptoms.

For the next four years I visited Michael every few months. Because my pattern of work was so unpredictable he let me call in on Saturday mornings if I was in the locality. At the time my godfather was still living in Canterbury and I combined my visits to him with my visits to the hospital.

THE END OF A LIFESTYLE

Because I visited on Saturdays I never saw the renal unit as it usually was, humming with activity. I would walk along the covered walkway to the main door and ring the bell. There is a forbidding notice telling all visitors to ring and wait before entering. If Michael was busy I might have a short wait, but before long I would be in his office having my blood pressure taken and answering any questions he might have. I noticed that if I had a heavy cold the blood in the urine would return. This, I later learned, was quite consistent with the kidney disease I had. Michael at one stage prescribed me some tablets to help with the anaemia the blood tests revealed. The anaemia must have crept up on me so slowly that I barely noticed I had less energy than before, and because I was still not convinced that I was ill, I must confess that I was not very conscientious about taking the pills. I felt that to commit myself to taking medication on a regular basis was an admission that I was ill. I did not want to admit that.

The ritual visits always included a blood test and that was the only thing I disliked. By and large my appointments to see Michael were more like social calls as we talked widely about my work and latest assignments.

I was at the time following a very punishing schedule. On my trips south to Orkney I would fill every available hour with work. I stayed in London with my aunt Mary in Upper Norwood and in Scotland with my sister in Fife or a bed-and-breakfast wherever I happened to be. I once worked out that I slept in a different place for eight nights running. Sometimes I would finish working with the Radio 4 'World Tonight' programme and catch the overnight bus to Glasgow to start a new day there.

It was apparent to Michael after a few visits that I had a condition called IgA nephropathy. To confirm the diagnosis, however, and to get some idea of its long-term progress I needed to have a renal biopsy. For that I needed to book into the hospital, something I did not relish.

In due course I was to get to know East Ward at the Kent and Canterbury well. My first visit, however, is not one which stands out in my mind. The only clear memory I have is of the biopsy itself. It was carried out in a side room of the ward and I lay on an examination table while a doctor, not Michael Goggin, pushed a special tool into my back. It was not so much a painful experience as one which produced a curious and unpleasant sensation inside. As I was on my front I could not see what was going on, but the procedure did not last long and soon the sample of kidney was snipped and extracted.

The biopsy confirmed the diagnosis: a particular form of kidney disease initially associated with infections of the upper respiratory tract and gastro-intestinal tract. It could have been set off by my Algerian bug or just been coincidental—there is no way of proving it either way. In my notes Michael Goggin has written, 'Evidence exists to link the disease with mesangial (glomerular) deposits of IgA containing immune complexes. There is a close association between active renal disease and the conditions above pointing to an interaction between viral and bacterial antigens with performed antibodies.'

As curious as I am about my illness I have not embarked on an exhaustive study of the science required to understand fully what is wrong with me. I am much more concerned with the practicalities of treatment and, particularly at that time, with the prognosis. How long would it be before my kidneys were likely to pack up?

At this stage Michael Goggin was reluctant to map out the future. When pressed he thought I might experience problems in my fifties. Being then only in my early thirties that seemed an age away and I continued my life much as before.

Between 1980, the year of the Algerian episode, and 1984, when my kidney disease began to dictate terms, I had three memorable trips abroad: to Zimbabwe, Lebanon and Nicaragua.

I went to Zimbabwe with John Newbury as producer. We

were collecting material for programmes about the country just after independence, when the scars of war were beginning to heal. A visit to two schools in the far south of the country I will never forget. Both had been in the thick of the fighting during the civil war and yet the staff were eager to forgive and rebuild their work, despite a severe shortage of money and equipment. One school was a Salvation Army foundation and the other was run by a remarkable husband-and-wife team who were Methodists. The man stamped his character on the school in an amazing way, despite being blind. At one point during the fighting the entire school had been marched across the nearby frontier by guerillas wanting to persuade the pupils to take up arms. In both places we witnessed a moving example of the triumph of faith over adversity. We met many very brave individuals facing odds no Christian would ever have to face in Britain.

We also travelled to the far north of the country and saw the Victoria Falls. I had earlier been to Zambia and had been disappointed not to see the Falls. To see the power of creation in such naked splendour is awe inspiring.

One curious feature of the Falls is that the spray from the thundering waters soaks the surrounding atmosphere and creates a tropical rain forest area, just half a mile wide, around the boundary of the great gorge.

We dined at the splendid hotel nearby and were served crocodile and chips. The crocodile had come from the crocodile farm close by where the reptiles were bred for their meat and skins. The stud beast was a huge fifteen-foot-long male called Big Daddy. The owners showed him to us with pride, boosting his reputation with the claim that he had in his lifetime eaten two people.

We also saw wild crocodiles and hippopotami in the Zambesi River, and on a journey south through the Wankie Game Park enjoyed some of the most amazing and precious sights on earth. At one point, we had to stop our vehicle to let a tribe of elephants cross the road ahead of us. There were some sixty animals of all sizes from the huge males, with their long tusks and enormous flapping ears, to babies who could barely keep up with the family. They were on their way to a water hole where we watched them wallowing in mud and blowing jets of water at each other with their trunks. Not long after, we stopped on the track again to admire a basking lion, less than six feet away.

My kidney problem only interfered in a minor way. One night I developed severe pains in one foot. It was very tender to stand on and for a while I hobbled. It was something with which I was familiar, having had attacks before, but it was only later I discovered it was connected to the progressive kidney failure. It was gout.

Gout is not something one readily admits to as it conjures up all sorts of images of eighteenth-century high life and over-indulgence in rich food and red wine. It is in fact a complaint often suffered by people who are never excessive in any of their drinking habits but who get an inflammation of the joints of the foot due to uric acid in the blood.

Having been awestruck by the wonders of creation in Zimbabwe and by the saintly demeanour of so many courageous individuals, my visit to Lebanon showed me the other side of life in full measure.

Being unable to fly direct to Beirut, as the airport was closed at the time, I took a plane to Tel Aviv and travelled from there to Jerusalem. As it was a Jewish holiday I had to wait in Israel before attempting to get in to Lebanon and took the opportunity of visiting the world's most famous city.

Some of my very earliest memories are of Sunday School and being shown pictures of the Holy Land. We were encouraged to draw pictures of flat-topped houses, donkeys, palm trees and people in local dress. I am told that I once up-dated the images by showing a man in Middle-Eastern head-dress flying an aeroplane which I called 'The Flight into Eygpt with

THE END OF A LIFESTYLE

Pontius the Pilot'. By and large, however, the authentic images stayed with me, reinforced by the vivid pictures of the Victorian artist Holman Hunt, whose series of water colours of the Holy Land we had bound as prints in a book.

With all these preconceived ideas to dispel I am amazed that I did not find Jerusalem disappointing. But the old walled city with its narrow streets and markets lived up to all expectations. I saw small boys holding donkey races in the Via Dolorosa. I saw gnarled, old Arab men with their heads covered in the traditional manner just like characters from a Holman Hunt print. I saw palm trees and flat-topped houses just as I had envisaged. Admittedly there were also wide-beamed American matrons carrying crosses and persistent salesmen who wanted me to buy postcards and souvenirs, and at the holiest site in all Christendom there was a kiosk selling plastic replica crowns of thorns.

To someone who has had a Christian upbringing, Jerusalem brings alive many of the Bible stories. Locations and places which seemed so far away and exotic become real places. To faith or spiritual curiosity is added historical credibility. Jerusalem is also the holy city for two other great religions, Judaism and Islam. The Islamic Dome of the Rock dominates the sky line and, as if to underline the tensions of the area and prepare me for what was to come in Lebanon, my way into the mosque was barred by armed guards. However, I did visit the Wailing Wall and saw the devotion of hundreds of Jews, heads covered, bobbing and bowing in prayer, at the sacred remnant of the old temple.

The intensity of their faith was brought home to me sharply when I foolishly ventured by car into an orthodox Jewish quarter on the Sabbath and had stones thrown at me by some angry young men.

To get to Beirut I had to fly to Cyprus and take the overnight ferry. It arrived in port full of refugees, and I saw one distraught woman having her pet dog confiscated by customs officials. I presume it was against regulations to bring dogs into Cyprus and it was due to be destroyed. I saw families sitting on bulging suitcases containing all their worldly possessions: hundreds of bemused people fleeing the fighting.

By contrast, the ferry into Beirut was almost completely empty. Two BBC colleagues whom I met in Cyprus decided to share a cabin at an exorbitant charge, while I opted to sleep on deck. Come the morning I knew I had made the better decision. Not only was the cabin swimming with water, but at dawn I saw one of the most extraordinary and chilling sights I had ever witnessed.

As the morning light increased I found we were sailing through the American fleet: huge, grey, silent ships of war with their powerful guns trained on the hills above the city. That night I was to learn why they were there, as American shells whistled overhead and the guns thundered out at sea.

My task in Lebanon was to compile a radio documentary that would provide a background to the conflict, trying to explain who was who when Christians or Shi'ites or Druze were mentioned in news bulletins. Through contacts I had been given in advance and people I met in Beirut, I was able to build up a picture of the protagonists and sketch some of the history of the conflict. It was, not unexpectedly, a difficult city in which to work. The electricity supply was spasmodic at best. The telephones were almost always out of commission, the streets were blocked with traffic and the debris of war, and the buildings were almost all damaged in some way. Little images stick in my mind; the dead cat left in the gutter outside the American University and the florist's shop that had been burned out inside but was still operating from the shell of a wrecked car on the pavement.

And yet in the midst of it all there were glimpses of normality. I went to one home full of the most beautiful decorations and furniture, an oasis of taste and culture in a desert of brutality and mindless hate. At one Christian hospital I met a bishop who spoke movingly and yet so wearily about life. He was living in a room at the hospital as his home was no longer habitable. He wore a spotless cream-coloured cassock and had a thick white beard. He appeared to me a holy man confused by evil.

Normally one is wary in a new city, not knowing its character and its dangers, but in Beirut I never felt wholly safe. Even in bed at night there was no real rest with the American guns firing. To be trapped in the city by circumstance, commitment or poverty must be unbearable. How Terry Waite and the other hostages must feel is beyond my imagination.

Yet the only direct danger I faced was in trying to leave the country. I needed to travel south to the Israeli border and from there hire a car to Tel Aviv.

I hitched a ride with a car taking American news footage to the frontier. It was driven very recklessly by a Lebanese driver who knew the way through the pot-holed streets and along the coastal road. As the journey progressed I realized that his speed was not recklessness but protection. More than once we heard the crack of gunfire as snipers took pot-shots at us.

Driving through the countryside we were stopped two or three times by armed men in battle dress. Which militia or army they were I do not know, but we were allowed through. In due course we reached the Israeli frontier. We were stopped by a soldier in casual dress about half a mile from the border post. We could go no further, he said: the border post was closed for the Sabbath. The driver appeared unworried and gave his package of news film to another man who was allowed through. I, however, was not, despite arguing that I had a flight to catch back to London from Tel Aviv. It is difficult to argue with a man with a gun and I had to retreat to the nearest village and book in at the hotel. There was only one room available and I had to share it with an American journalist who was also trying to cross to Israel. That night was disturbed yet again, this time by an all-night wedding feast downstairs.

The next morning we visited the United Nations post and asked if they could help get us through. They were not surprised to see us: it seems the Israeli border was notoriously difficult to cross at that point. However, there was a way, so we gratefully accepted a ride in a United Nations truck which had the right to travel across. Once back in Israel I had a mad dash for the airport but missed the plane. With a programme deadline looming I called London, rebooked on another airline and came home via Amsterdam.

I sometimes look back with alarm and wonder what would have happened if my kidneys had decided to cease functioning when I was in some place like Beirut where medical services were basic and easy transport back to Britain impossible. At that stage I was not taking my health seriously, despite my regular visits to Canterbury. It seemed inconceivable that I would one day be ill.

In November 1983, just two months after my return from the Middle East, I found myself on a plane to Nicaragua to record a profile of Daniel Ortega, then emerging as the new president of the country. I had been to Central America before, but this time I was going to a country ruled by a left-wing rather than a right-wing regime. I was very fortunate in having as a guide a friend who had worked for the 'Sunday' programme and who was now in the country as a freelance journalist.

Despite its reputation as a war-torn country, I felt Nicaragua to be safe. It had a delightful provincial feel to it, more like a small town than a nation state. The Sandinistas, the revolutionaries who ruled the country, were much in evidence in Managua. Indeed, it is said that when Daniel Ortega took power, he declared that he did not want an office in the government building but would be content travelling the country in his jeep, meeting the people.

One evening I was taken to a small seaside town on the Pacific coast famed for its seafood. Along the sea front were dozens of makeshift huts surrounded by tables where the local fish were cooked and served. But as we called at each hut we were told the same story; 'Sorry, no fish today.' It seemed curious that this fishing town should not be able to provide the basic ingredients of a meal. However, we soon realized what was happening. The entire fishing fleet had been commandeered to ferry arms ashore from Russian ships in the bay.

Before meeting Daniel Ortega, I met his wife. I learned, to my surprise, that she had been a pupil at a girls' boarding school in Somerset. She talked graphically of the revolution and of the ousting of the dictator Somoza. She recalled how one night the Sandinista command was staying a few miles out of Managua and heard an aircraft overhead. One of them joked that that was Somoza leaving the country. The next morning they discovered it was true and shortly afterwards entered the capital city in triumph.

We met Daniel Ortega in a small inner room in the government building. He was wearing military fatigues and welcomed us quite informally. He is about my age and is as far from the American image of the bombastic Communist as you could imagine. He was, if anything, rather shy and diffident. I found him impressive and honest with an ordinariness denied many people in power.

There was one occasion when I found my experience in Lebanon stood me in good stead. I was talking to a Nicaraguan military leader and asking him about the war with the Contras. He was very reluctant to answer any questions. I asked him why he was being so cautious. 'You don't know what it is like to be on the receiving end of American gun fire,' he said.

'Oh yes I do,' I said. 'Only two months ago I was being fired at by the whole American Mediterranean fleet.' He immediately became more friendly and forthcoming.

My trip to Nicaragua was, however, marred by headaches which were to herald the final kidney failure. I remember one evening having dinner with the ITN correspondent Jon Snow and having a huge steak. Steaks were very cheap and I took advantage of the fact. That night I suffered from sickness and headaches. The high protein intake had overloaded the dwindling kidney function and pushed up the blood pressure to an uncomfortable level—not that I realized at that stage what was happening.

My diary, or more precisely my appointments book, for the first four months of 1984 shows my life to have been the usual round of hectic working trips interspersed with journeys home to Orkney. At the beginning of the year we moved from Rousay to Orkney mainland, to a new house called 'Kelda' in the parish of Birsay. We had moorland around us and a marvellous view of a loch from the kitchen window. It was a practical move. We were released from the financial burdens of the huge old house on the island and my journey to and from home was easier in that I no longer had a ferry crossing to Rousay. The children ceased being weekly boarders and went on a daily basis to school in Stromness. On the hill behind the house we could see the huge wind-turbine built experimentally to provide some of the islands' power and now joined by an even more substantial machine. It was a far more comforting sight than the insidious Dounreay Fast reactor on the other side of the Pentland Firth.

During our time in Orkney, when I could I worked as near to home as possible, and Dounreay provided a number of stories. One assignment involved researching the case of the missing fuel pins for 'Panorama' and the *Daily Mail*. One consequence of that story was that I was contacted by a man who had been involved in a radiation incident at Dounreay and was now dying of cancer. My diary reminds me that he died early in 1984 and we were waiting for the inquest to be held. It was inexplicably delayed for many weeks.

I remember sitting with him at his home before he died. He was weak and thin from cancer and very pale. A photograph of him showed him as a full-faced ebullient character; now he was brought physically low by illness. But his mind was sharp, and in his younger days he had kept meticulous records which he was able to produce to show what had happened to him at the nuclear plant. As much as I was dreading the day when I felt my freedom would be curtailed by being tied to a kidney machine, I did reflect that I was lucky to have an illness which could be held in check and would not inevitably condemn me to early death.

That year, 1984, I also recorded a long interview with the Prince of Wales about the Prince's Trust and some of the projects it was supporting. I hope Welsh royalists will not be too shocked to learn that in the lavatory at Kensington palace, framed and hanging on the wall, is the illuminated scroll of the freedom of the City of Cardiff.

I suppose in some ways I was a workaholic. I certainly spent more time at work than at home and the family still complains, 'Oh, you were never there!' My colleagues found it intriguing that I managed to live in Orkney and yet be in so many places at the right time—an invaluable asset for a journalist. I contributed regularly to the BBC Scotland output, both radio and television, and would often amaze my fellow journalists back at base by ringing from some far-away location which just happened to be in the news.

This lifestyle came to an end on my birthday, 14 April 1984. It was a Saturday and I had an appointment with Michael Goggin at 11 a.m. The weeks before, my headaches had become more frequent. I recall that on one occasion I was at Scrabster waiting for the Orkney ferry to cross when I could barely see because my head was so bad.

This I duly reported to Michael Goggin and he took my blood pressure. It was sky high. Treatment had to start. It was not initially on a kidney machine but by means of a controlled diet. My protein intake was to be radically reduced and my fluid intake raised to 3 litres a day. I was given a list of forbidden foods. I was not at that stage told about restricting my potassium intake but, judging from the list I was given, a potassium restriction must have been included in the diet. I was told to eat no more than 3 ounces of meat, or a little more of fish, and to avoid instant coffee, chocolate, banana, red wine, fresh fruit, eggs and cheese. I was told about cooking vegetables well and draining them, but curiously no mention was made of potatoes or tomatoes or mushrooms. I continued to eat them, as their protein content was low and protein was what I had been told to avoid. Now I know these foods to be high in potassium and a lot worse in many instances than chocolate biscuits.

The dietician was very friendly, but perhaps I misunderstood her. Or perhaps she made the assumption that no British person can live without potatoes and so the diet must be amended accordingly. On reflection I now feel very strongly that the exact nature and purpose of the diet should have been spelt out far more clearly and far more information given than just a set of good foods and bad foods.

I also started taking tablets for blood pressure and kept to the regime very closely, as I soon knew if I had forgotten to take one of the prescribed anti-hypertensives.

I was also introduced to special low-protein foods, available from chemists on prescription. I would collect boxes of low protein pastas, biscuits and tins of bread from the doctor's dispensary in Orkney.

The pasta was palatable and, cooked with an imaginative sauce, was very filling. The biscuits were too often over sweet, but the wafer biscuits were good for filling what now seemed like a permanent hunger gap. The bread was edible if toasted. However, the high calorie drink it was suggested I take was quite revolting. It looked like engine oil and tasted of molten plastic. I had always enjoyed good food, and one of the ironies of the situation was that just as I was put on the diet I was approached by *The Good Food Guide* to be one of their part-time inspectors.

I found it very hard to adjust to the discipline of ill health and it took me a few months before I was able to say I was keeping strictly to the diet. On two occasions I must admit I stretched it beyond its credible bounds.

Shortly after my April meeting with Michael Goggin I was due to go to the Greek Islands on a press trip. In the Greek *tavernas* I was very good in steering clear of meat in quantity and red wine but I did eat more vegetables than I should have done. And in May I flew to Toronto to spend a week with Florence Tim Oi Li, the remarkable Chinese lady who had been ordained as the first Anglican woman priest. I had been asked to write a book about her. In the mornings and afternoons we talked and I recorded her reminiscences. At lunchtimes we visited one of the many Chinese restaurants in Toronto's Chinatown and Miss Li introduced me to the delights of Chinese cuisine. For one delightful, naughty week I was an unashamed dietary backslider.

It has been one of the privileges of my work, and I can think of no better word than privilege, to have met so many truly courageous and saintly people. Florence Li was born into a society which was still feudal. The Empress was still on the throne and her aunts had been of the generation of girls who had their feet bound to make them small, with the result that they had to be carried about by maidservants.

Florence, however, was brought up a Christian. She became a priest during the Second World War when she was administering to a congregation which had no access to the sacraments. She was called by Bishop Hall to come and see him and made a dangerous journey through the Japanese lines. Bishop Hall ordained her a priest because she was the best-qualified person to provide a sacramental ministry to her isolated congregation. His decision caused enormous problems elsewhere in the Anglican communion but Florence Li was unaware of the debate and continued her work in China whenever she could, lost to the outside world. Only when she was retired and China was opening up did people from the

West meet her again. She came to Toronto to join some of her family who were living there.

My trip to the Greek islands had a spiritual side too. It included a visit to Patmos, the island of St John where the Book of Revelation was written.

The island is visited by tourists, but not in great numbers. So when I arrived at the monastery at the top of the hill it was as a pilgrim. There were no motor vehicles around, few souvenirs to be bought, and a monastery that was quite uncommercialized. It was as if I had gone back eight hundred years into history. A monk announced afternoon prayer by walking the courtyards and corridors of the monastery rhythmically beating a large piece of resonant wood which looked like an aeroplane propeller. I was the only outsider present and was invited to join the monks at their office. We sat in a darkened chapel, the smell and smoke from incense and candles filling the air. Slowly the ancient music of prayer began and I sat transfixed. As my eyes became accustomed to the gloom I began to see ornate golden icons covering the walls, somewhat blackened by smoke and time but nevertheless clear images of Christ and the saints. I only knew I was in the twentieth century because two of the monks wore spectacles.

That summer we went as a family to Sweden. It was mostly as a holiday, but I had a programme to make for the English service of Swedish radio. By that time I knew when dialysis was likely to start. From my regular visits to Canterbury and from the blood tests taken, Michael Goggin was able to give a count-down to D-day. I knew that our Swedish holiday was likely to be the last time we could get away together as a family for more than two or three days.

His forecast was remarkably accurate. 1984 ended with me being given an appointment as an in-patient at Canterbury to have the veins in my wrist prepared for the inevitable dialysis. So on 9 January 1985 I reported to the sister on East Ward for my fistula operation.

3

A NEW ROUTINE

Having a fistula constructed in the wrist as a means of access for the dialysis needles is a relatively simple procedure. It can be done under a local anaesthetic and I was insistent that I did not want to have an extended stay in hospital to recover from a general anaesthetic.

However, I was not prepared for the breakdown in communication which ensued and from which I learned a number of valuable lessons about how to look after my best interests as a patient.

On the morning of the operation someone put a notice on my bed 'Nil orally', the usual sign that the patient in question was about to have a general anaesthetic. There was a mistake, I told the nurse who refused to give me any breakfast. I was having my operation under a local. No one took much notice of my protestations until I pointed out that the sign at the foot of the bed contradicted the instructions given to me by the consultant that I had to drink up to 3 litres of fluid a day. A junior doctor was called and her solution was to put me on a drip. I should have refused but as a new patient one is peculiarly powerless. In due course Michael Goggin came on his ward round and I explained the confusion to him. He immediately confirmed that I was to be given a local anaesthetic and the drip was removed.

I dressed myself in a surgical gown and in due course was wheeled along the corridor to the place where patients wait and worry. After a while I was wheeled through to an anteroom where the anaesthetist injected my armpit with I know not what and asked if I felt any sensation in my hand. On the second pin-prick a jolt of pain shot through my thumb. When I reported that he was satisfied.

Ten minutes later I was in the theatre having my left arm painted in an oriental yellow paint, an antiseptic I was told. The rest of me was covered in a green sheet. My view was 90 per cent green sheet, 9 per cent overhead lights and 1 per cent the bright red ear of the surgeon working away.

The operation itself was no worse than going to the dentist. I am short-sighted and because I was denied the use of my glasses during the procedure, I was spared the sight of the gruesome cold steel of the theatre.

It all took about three quarters of an hour. I felt the incision and the stitching, but it did not hurt. The boredom was relieved only by a faulty blood pressure gauge on my right arm which, at one stage, blew up like a balloon.

Once the operation was over and I was back in the recovery room my fistula was listened to with a stethoscope. A third-year nurse tried and heard nothing. She called another nurse: he heard very little. I was wheeled back to the ward not knowing if the operation had been successful or not. If it had been a failure I would have to return to the theatre. When the surgeon came to look, however, he was satisfied and it was only a matter of waiting to be discharged with a heavily-bandaged arm.

Once the stitches were out and the wound healed I felt rather proud of my fistula. I would invite people to listen to it (it made a loud swishing noise) or feel it buzz. My doctor in

A NEW ROUTINE

Orkney had never seen one before and was fascinated. The fistula has served me well. After four years of constant use the veins are all in good shape and my left arm is not a mass of lumps and bruises like the arms of many renal patients.

The first six months of 1985 were busy, but not as hectic as before. One of my regular commitments was as a reporter on 'The World at One' and 'PM' programmes and it suited me well to travel south for a week or two, staying with Aunt Mary, and then travelling home again. In my time journeying to and from Orkney I must have used every available form of transport. I drove the whole length of the country on a number of occasions, went by bus, train, plane and even once by sailing ship via the western isles.

As 1985 progressed I began to feel increasingly tired yet unable to relax. My legs twitched as an unbearable tension built up. I found my concentration waning and by June I must have been very ill. I was writing a book at the time about David Jenkins, Bishop of Durham, and found I could not work for more than half an hour at a time. Much of the day was spent lying down or sitting in the round greenhouse in the garden which trapped the northern sun.

It soon became clear to everyone except me that I needed to go back to Canterbury and start dialysing. It was the last thing I wanted to do. I knew I was not going to get better any other way but I hated the idea of closing a chapter of my life and starting a new one full of the unknown. A curious and irrational fear which bothered me was that once I started dialysing I would no longer be able to pee. It was a groundless fear, as urine can still be produced in small amounts by diseased kidneys.

At the end of June Helen persuaded me to see the doctor, who in turn persuaded me to go south for treatment. Even if I had not been a patient of Michael Goggin I would still have needed to travel south as Orkney had no renal facilities. Had I known what I do today I could have gone south to Aberdeen and there been started on CAPD (Continuous Ambulatory Peritoneal Dialysis) before returning home.

At the time the only option seemed to be to travel to Canterbury and be admitted to East Ward. My flight to Aberdeen and on to London was booked. It was even arranged that at Aberdeen and London I would be met by British Airways staff with a wheelchair. Ever stubborn, I carefully avoided that ignominy. I was met by friends at Heathrow and next day set off by train to Canterbury.

I knew I was about to start a new life. I knew I was not to see the northern isles for many years. It was a little like starting a new job or even a new school. I felt sick with the illness and with apprehension.

I was welcomed by the sister on East Ward like an old friend. I was booked in and fussed over and before long I found the routine of the ward reassuring. I did not have to worry about travel or the next meal. I was, however, growing increasingly anxious about my work, and my book on David Jenkins in particular. I had all the research material with me and spent a few days trying to work in the open ward. When one of the single rooms became free I was moved in. I do not now recall how long I was in hospital. Days seem to merge into each other in my memory. I recall the endless sleepless nights when I could not lie still for more than a minute or two at a time and had to walk the corridor to get any respite from the muscular tensions caused by the poisons in my body.

In short bursts I would work on my book. The illness did not help me tackle the abstruse theology of the famous bishop but I battled on. Sometimes the inability to relax made me want to scream and cry. There were times when I felt very low and alone. The family was eight hundred miles away and I could only call them from the ward pay-phone when it was not being used by others.

I was not entirely restricted to the ward. If I felt up to it I could leave the hospital and go and see friends. I went to see

Martin and Christian Claridge, who also visited me on the ward, and Roger and Sandy Mitchell, friends of many years standing who were to let me stay at their cottage just outside Canterbury to allow me to qualify for treatment as a local resident. Some days I sat outside the ward in the sun. It was a hot summer. From time to time the heat set fire alarms off and fire engines raced up to the hospital from the town.

Despite wrestling with matters theological in the course of my writing I felt too ill to have many deep thoughts of my own. If I had died then it would have been a strange anti-climax to life. After a week or two in hospital all passion and hope had left me and I just survived. I drank what I was told to drink, measured my output, reported the results. I was woken every morning for a cup of tea and fifteen minutes later, after a brief and welcome sleep, I would be woken up again for my temperature and blood pressure to be taken. Then after another doze it was time for tablets and by the time breakfast arrived I felt as if I had been subjected to a night of sleep-deprivation torture.

One day I was visited by a retired bishop whom I knew through my godfather. As he was about to go after a chat, no doubt about the family and cricket and perhaps David Jenkins, he placed his hands on my head and said a prayer. It was quite unexpected and I believe spontaneous on his part. The Christian ministry of the laying on of hands was something I knew about in theory but had never expected to be applied to me. I was in an open ward and I think initially I felt a bit embarrassed. But that feeling did not last long as the prayer was short and the gesture did not attract attention. I remember it calmed me and it was a moment I looked back on many times as I lay awake at night. It was not healing in the sense that it did not miraculously cause my kidneys to recover, but it was healing in that it gave me the seed of hope I needed. Over the subsequent weeks I relied on that seed of hope and in time saw it grow.

At one stage Michael Goggin contemplated starting me on

peritoneal dialysis. This would have involved having a tube stuck in my tummy and my peritoneal cavity filled with dialysate solution. The thought of having a tube permanently stuck inside me filled me with dread and I said so. Nothing came of the idea. I was by now feeling so ill that I wanted to start dialysing. I had gone past the fear of what dialysis might mean to my lifestyle: I just wanted some treatment to relieve the symptoms of kidney failure. I was getting short of breath and my body was starting to retain fluid. I weighed a whole 10 kilograms more than I do now because my body was retaining over 2 gallons or 10 litres of excess water.

Days went by without anything much happening. I understand that behind the scenes Michael Goggin was in the middle of a battle for resources. To accept a new patient onto the haemodialysis programme is to commit the hospital, or health authority, to a massive annual expenditure for an indefinite period.

One evening Mark, the nurse who was number two in charge of the renal unit, came to see me. 'Tomorrow,' he said, 'we will start your dialysis.' He outlined what would happen and I had all night to think about it. I believe it was around midday on July 16 that I was taken to the renal unit.

I can still recall my first impression of the unit. Although I now go there and feel it is familiar territory, that first feeling of shock, fear and amazement lingers on. The impression is not just built up by what one sees—the ten beds or chairs with patients allowing their blood to be taken by tube from their arms through the workings of the kidney machine and back. There is also the noise of the unit—the constant sound of pumps and the occasional sound of alarms. Most evocative of all is the smell. It is an all pervasive and unique odour which is so strong it clings to your clothes and stays with you when you have left the hospital.

The ward sister Daphne Tulloch put the needles into my arm for the first time. I was on a relatively gentle dialyser contained in what was known as a pot, a bubbling glass bucket of dialysis solution inside which there was a coil through which my blood circulated. On my first visit to the unit I did not take in much about the machinery. I was content to be treated. I was on the machine for four hours, two hours less than I dialyse now, but it seemed like an age. At the end of the afternoon I felt worse than ever. My blood pressure was high and I felt weak and sick. I could barely walk and all I wanted to do was sleep. One thing I did notice was that the tensions in my muscles which prevented me from relaxing had eased.

Just as I was about to go to sleep I was told that my family was outside—my parents and my sister. My memory of events is hazy but I do know that visitors were the last thing I needed. I felt, and must have looked, so dreadful that I wanted a night's sleep to recover. I sent the message that I would love to see them in the morning, but before I knew what was happening there they were in my room asking me how I was feeling. As grateful as I was for their concern I do wish they had waited until the morning when I was feeling much more able to be communicative and to enjoy their company.

From July 16 onwards I wrote a big 'D' in my diary every Tuesday and Friday. The second time I dialysed I was encouraged to put my own needles in and have done so ever since. As the weeks went by I became more and more familiar with the machine and it became less of an ogre.

My diet was also changed, my fluid intake cut by two thirds and my protein intake raised by a little. Potassium was still to be avoided and it was spelt out why: excess potassium causes the heart to stop, sometimes without warning.

With every meal I had to take a small red-and-green capsule called an alucap. This is a phosphate binder and if I take it I do not have to be so careful about monitoring the phosphates in my diet. Uncontrolled intake of phosphates can lead to long-term problems with bones in a renal patient. I now, however, take a calcium-based phosphate binder. I asked for the change because I was concerned about the long-term build-up of aluminium in the brain, which can cause dementia.

There used to be a notice in the renal unit saying alucaps had to be taken ten minutes after a meal. When I pointed this out to the dietician, just after she had told me to take the tablet ten minutes before a meal for maximum effect, the notice in the renal unit was quietly changed.

The unit is run according to some very strict rules. These are mostly designed to prevent the spread of hepatitis. Special shoes and clothes must be worn. No one can cross the barrier into the unit unless they have had a blood test and been declared hepatitis free. Objects such as newspapers and books can be taken in to the unit but not out again. After use they have to be put into a bag marked 'infected waste'. The value of these rules has been proved by the fact that Canterbury has been hepatitis free for a very long time. Curiously there are some anomalies. Patients are encouraged to reuse bandages and these can be brought in and out of the unit many times.

One of the problems involved in operating strictly by the rule book is that when something happens which is not anticipated it is sometimes not believed. For instance, most dialysis patients find that on haemodialysis their blood pressure drops. Curiously, I found that mine went up, at least in the initial months. For a long while no one believed me and people would insist on adjusting the pressures of the machine and making matters worse.

The relationship that develops between staff and patients is an unusual one. Everyone gets to know everyone else very well. Friendships develop, but a feeling persists that the staff believe they have an authority. Any undermining of that authority is resented. And yet to my mind it ought to be a relationship of equals. The staff have an area of specialist knowledge and we, as patients, are their clients. It is certainly essential to my well-being that I feel that I am in control of my destiny. I remember times when alarms sounded on a machine to indicate a problem and a young nurse would come over and say, 'Who's causing trouble today then?'

One of the battles I had was about home dialysis. According to the rules of the unit a new patient, after a few months training, would have a dialysis machine installed in his or her home. This I did not want, but it was assumed that when we bought a house down south, as we were doing by the new year of 1985, a machine would be installed. The reason I did not want to dialyse at home was that, according to the rules, I would have had to dialyse three times a week at set times in the evening. This would have played havoc with my work. Secondly, I did not want the family tied down by my illness. And thirdly, I wanted to be able to live at home, forget about the treatment and not be constantly reminded that I was a kidney patient by the very presence of the machine in the house. On one occasion the home dialysis administrator even went to look at a house we were thinking of buying to size it up for a machine.

In January 1986 I started dialysing at Keycol, a minimal-care satellite unit. There, four patients dialyse at one go with the help of two assistants. We dialyse twice a week during the day. I did some research and discovered that it was cheaper for patients to dialyse at such units than to go to the expense of kitting out a home. But the pressure on me to become a home dialysis patient only lifted when we bought a house at Conyer near Sittingbourne which was clearly not suitable for the installation of a home unit.

If one has to dialyse anywhere I can think of no better place than Keycol. At the time of writing there are four of us dialysing every Tuesday and Friday: Sandra, Stephen, Gerald and myself. The AKAs (artificial kidney assistants) who help us are Cyn, Wendy and Eva. Cyn and Eva alternate but Wendy is there almost every time. It is a good atmosphere and we all get on very well. Before his transplant one of my fellow patients was a high Tory called Bernard who was ragged unmercifully at election time. Then there was Brian, who also had a transplant; Michael, who left for another unit when he got married; and Dick who was woken up by Michael Goggin one day as he was dialysing and told to get up to Guys Hospital with all speed as a kidney awaited him.

A Keycol day for me begins at about 8 a.m. when I arrive at the unit, which is housed in a wooden building in the grounds of an old people's home near Sittingbourne, to set up the machine. Usually Eva or Cyn is there and has turned on the water and turned up the heating. Setting up the machine involves threading one of the long plastic lines through the pump and connecting it to the dialyser tube and then taking another line, joining it to the other end of the dialyser and connecting it up to the machine alarms. It looks a complicated procedure but I am now so used to it that it comes as second nature. As a result I do not always concentrate on the task as I should and by the end have forgotten some vital ingredient. Once assembled the whole system has to be primed with a saline solution and clamped off at either end, and then it is time to prepare the pack. This is a sterilized pack containing swabs and paper towels, to which are added the two hollow dialysing needles, a syringe, a small needle and a syringe for the local anaesthetic.

There are various other preparations to be made and in all it takes about half to three-quarters of an hour. Then, with some help from Cyn, Eva or Wendy, I stick the needles into my vein, connect them up to the lines and turn the machine on. From time to time the machine alarms, if the flow of blood from the vein is in any way impeded or if air gets into the lines carrying the dialysate solution. Sometimes the machine is temperamental and a technician from Canterbury comes over to put it right.

The six hours on dialysis pass fairly quickly. To begin with I read the newspaper and then we are all brought some toast and something to drink for breakfast. I usually have a pile of work with me, in a large plastic bag to protect it from blood spills, and we also have a television. My only complaint is that the radio is tuned to Radio 1 and Gerald hums along! We bring our own lunch and I sometimes bring left-overs from the night before to be heated up in the microwave.

At the end of six hours we follow the reverse procedure of turning the machine off and removing the needles and bandaging the arm. By four o'clock in the afternoon I am normally away. I am not usually feeling at my best immediately after dialysis and ideally like to go home and sleep. This is not often possible. Once I counted ten phone calls between returning home and six o'clock. Quite often I have to go straight from Keycol up to London, or even further afield. It is not unknown for me to dash madly from dialysis to the airport to catch a plane for America.

Michael Goggin and the renal unit have been very helpful. Should I need to change my dialysis days to suit my work schedule they willingly agree. Only once have I ever delayed returning to dialyse, and that by only a day, on a trip to make a film in the south of France.

I am not sure that I am a good patient. I am certainly a reluctant one. I argue and have a mind of my own which sometimes exasperates those in the medical profession more used to compliant patients. But I believe it has been shown statistically that the difficult patients are those who thrive best. And on that basis I will continue to be, and recommend other patients to be, someone who takes nothing at face value and tries to stay in control as much as possible.

4

SMALL MIRACLES

There were times when I lay dialysing in the renal unit at Canterbury and wondered if I would ever work again. I supposed I could always make a living writing or drawing, but would I ever again be able to travel and go to interesting and new locations and meet with the people who made the news?

The spirit was very willing but the flesh was frustratingly weak. My blood pressure was erratic. Some days, usually on and just after dialysing, it would shoot right up, giving me headaches and making me feel sick; at other times it would drop so savagely that I could hardly stand up straight. I found everything I did tired me and the thought of working a twelve-hour day seemed impossible.

For much of the summer I was quite sure I would never travel again. The idea of working as a reporter for the BBC seemed absurd. I would look around the renal unit and see fellow patients whose hopes and horizons seemed so limited by their condition that they appeared to do little more in life than just survive from one day of treatment to the next. It did not occur to me until much later that the patients I saw around me were not representative of the whole. They were the acute cases or those with special problems. Unseen, because they were dialysing at home or in minimal-care units, were many more of Canterbury's renal patients who were getting on with life very well. I was not helped by reading a booklet produced by the British Kidney Patients Association. It had been designed, no doubt, to encourage new patients but I found it most depressing. It consisted of essays by patients on how they managed to get away from home and go on holiday. They all seemed to make such a fuss about doing things that were so trivial and gave the impression that to get away for a week in a caravan on a site by the seaside involved planning of military proportions. The more I read the more I concluded that I would have to forget foreign travel and indeed any form of reporting away from base. I concluded that I would now have to get used to the idea that I was entering the last phase of my life. All the excitement, I decided, was now behind me. I would have to live on my memories.

I was not initially encouraged even by returning gently to work. I started again with the features section of 'The World at One' and one of my first assignments involved meeting a potential interviewee at a London club for lunch. What he must have made of me I do not know, for my blood pressure was so low I could barely concentrate on the conversation and had to find an excuse to sit down at every possible opportunity. He was an elderly gentleman who appeared himself very spruce and fit.

Gradually, however, I found ways of coping. At the end of August I found myself doing a feature on football crowds. It involved travelling to the Wimbledon football team's training ground and interviewing the manager and some of the players. Travelling out of London, organizing the interviews and getting back to Broadcasting House required a lot of effort but I am sure no one I met that day suspected I was a kidney patient. That was the way I wanted it.

My first trip away from the south-east of England involved

a drive to the west country. Caroline came with me to see a fascinating and ambitious project in Dorset involving the renovation of an historic home as a centre for young people to come and study Shakespeare. It was a September Saturday and Caroline had just started at a new school. We had decided it would be best for her to start her 'O' level courses at an English school rather than have to switch from the Scottish to the English system mid-stream. David and Helen stayed behind in Orkney for David to complete his final year in the sixth form at Stromness. Caroline's school was her mother's old school under a different name, and for the duration she was to stay with her grandparents in Surrey. Meanwhile I was living in Canterbury on dialysis days, in London with Aunt Mary during the rest of the week and in Surrey at the weekends. This was our way of life until the purchase of our new house down south was complete and we could all be together again as a family.

The trip to Dorset went very smoothly and again I got through the day without anyone needing to know I was in anything but normal health. My confidence was returning. I still, however, needed to prove to myself that I could cope with even the most demanding of assignments.

As it happened, a week after our trip to Dorset I had the chance to find out. I had been asked to investigate the strange phenomenon of the moving statue of Ballinspittle for the Radio 4 programme 'Soundings'.

Ballinspittle is a small village in county Cork in Eire. In July 1985 a mother and daughter had reported that the statue of the Virgin Mary in the roadside grotto just outside the village had appeared to move. As the summer passed more and more people reported seeing the statue move and sightings of moving Madonnas were reported from other parts of Ireland. By September there had been over thirty similar stories, many of which had been embellished to include statues which not only moved but raised their arms, talked and even walked.

Enormous crowds gathered at the grottos to see the phenomena and on one night alone at Ballinspittle a crowd of fifteen thousand was reported and sixty-two buses were counted parked in the lane, along with five fish-and-chip vans to provide the physical sustenance to complement the spiritual. Not surprisingly, the documentary I was asked to make was titled 'Madonna Mania'.

Admittedly the Irish Republic is not as foreign as Zambia or Nicaragua but it was a country I had not visited before. I knew the north of Ireland well, but the south is distinctly non-British in feel and I was venturing into new territory. I needed to get to know the village, see and judge the statue for myself, consult scientific and theological experts, record my material and return to Britain in a space of less than three days in order to get back to Canterbury in time for my next dialysis. From experience I knew I was in for a hard physical and intellectual challenge. As I waited for the late-morning flight from Heathrow to Cork to take off I had time to wonder and worry if I would manage.

Thanks to the village postmaster, the parish priest, the local bishop and the Department of Applied Psychology at University College, Cork, I returned according to schedule with material for a programme which gave a plausible explanation for all the extraordinary events.

And extraordinary they certainly were. On the first evening I drove out from Cork along the winding lanes to Ballinspittle. It was a grey, drizzling day and I hardly expected to see many people out in the open in such weather. However, the lanes around the village were packed with parked cars and buses. In the sloping field opposite the grotto there must have been over a thousand of the faithful. The fish-and-chip vans were doing brisk business. The people stood murmuring the rosary, accompanying the sound of a prayer leader over a makeshift loud speaker. The statue was three or four feet tall and was set in a small, well-tended garden. When I arrived it was almost dark and the statue was lit by a halo of light bulbs. From time to time someone in the crowd would exclaim, 'She moved!' and describe excitedly to his or her neighbour what the statue had just appeared to do. Sometimes there would be gasps of surprise from some of the devotees and occasionally someone would offer a special prayer for a sick friend or relative out loud.

I recorded the sounds of the evening and then stood on the hillside about thirty yards away from the statue and watched. I concentrated on the figure in the distance and waited. After a few minutes the statue of the Virgin Mary did indeed appear to move. She did not raise her arms or try to communicate but the figure which had for a while been totally motionless and inanimate gave the impression of swaying from side to side. Being of a somewhat sceptical disposition I did not immediately shout out that I had seen a miracle but concluded that what I had seen was far more consistent with the theories of the applied psychologists at University College, Cork, than with divine or any other supernatural intervention. Their explanation was based on experiments they had carried out which showed how people in the dark moved and swayed unwittingly. The team leader explained the happenings in this way.

'When people weren't given visual contact with their environment then their movements were a lot less controlled and they weren't able to stay still and moved and swayed about a lot. So what could be happening at Ballinspittle is that when you are there at twilight you haven't got visual contact with your immediate surroundings. As is usual you are going to start swaying about on your feet, perhaps your neck will start trembling as you might have been looking up for too long and on the back of your eye you will see the image of that little lit statue on top of the hill. You will see that image moving. Because people are not aware that it is themselves who are moving, they will interpret that movement as being the statue.'

Yet at Ballinspittle people have reported seeing more than

just movement of the statue. One man I spoke to described how the face of Mary would sometimes change to that of Christ and others reported seeing the cloak billow out. The University College, Cork, team however had a scientific answer.

'We know from a lot of experiments that have been done in psychology since the 1950s that if someone looks at a hazy image, an ambiguous image, then they are going to interpret what they see, they are going to make up their own best guesses as to what they are looking at. We also know that if you stare at something for any length of time your eyes will become hazy. So if you stare at a statue for a couple of minutes without blinking your eyes too much that statue is going to become rather hazy in outline to you and you will not be seeing the fine detail, and it is very possible that you might start to interpret what you see according to what you want to see.'

On investigation it transpired that people had seen the statue move before but until the summer of 1985 no one had made a big issue of these optical illusions. Why then had Madonna Mania broken out when it did?

The shrewd postmaster Daniel Costello made this observation: 'People have shown an interest in the supernatural when times have been hard. In times of prosperity it's a case of God is in his heaven and all is right with the world, but then in times of recession, as now, when their whole way of life is upset, it is time to look to a more supernatural approach to their dilemma. I have heard that after the war in Italy, three hundred statues moved and whether that was the Virgin in heaven trying to console her people or what, I don't know.'

The Roman Catholic Church always approaches supernatural sightings with some caution. It likes to keep control of the spiritual lives of the faithful and to guide them in the way it sees fit and does not like to be side-tracked by what it would see as ephemeral manifestations of excessive folk piety.

I went to see the local bishop, Michael Murphy, Bishop of Cork and Ross. He had not himself been to Ballinspittle to see the statue, not wishing to lend events there a stamp of church approval. However, he confirmed that in Ireland that summer a new excitement had returned to church life and much good had followed from people meeting at the grottos.

'They are very prayerful gatherings, very devotional, and I also know that the effect has been very good for quite a number of people. Direct divine or supernatural intervention in the affairs of men is extremely rare and for that reason one has to approach any alleged appearances or movements with caution. It is common sense that one would first of all want to be sure that all possible natural explanations are exhausted before the church would decide there had been some divine intervention. There have been similar instances in the past and as you know it is reaching almost epidemic proportions at the moment, sightings of this kind. I think that by waiting things might clarify themselves. If we had to set up a commission for all the reported movements of statues and encounters with the Blessed Virgin we would be working overtime.'

If the bishop was not going to rush in and endorse the sightings as of God, he had to have some way of explaining why there was, to use his own expression 'almost an epidemic' of moving statues.

'First of all we have had a very bad summer, a very depressing summer. People haven't been able to go to the beach, haven't been able to go swimming. It must have been awful for people in caravans with children. And here is this thing suddenly reported in the media which people have seen. People's curiosity was naturally aroused and Ballinspittle was a place to go to. The other thing of course is that we are living in a very difficult time in Ireland. We have very high unemployment, which is a very depressing factor—specially for the individuals who are unemployed. It is very, very serious. Within the church there is a certain questioning of accepted values, matters of faith; and then too there is the threat of nuclear destruction, felt by young people very much I think. They wonder if it is worthwhile putting in all the work to prepare for a profession. People generally may be in need of some sign of reassurance.'

Bishop Murphy accepted that the sightings contained in them a message for the leaders of the church. The people of Ireland, he said, were hungry for a spirituality of their own.

'Since Vatican II there has been great emphasis on the intellectual side of things, discussion on various matters pertaining to the church and belief. Some of this may well have passed over the heads of people. Not enough attention was paid to the emotional side of religion and certainly there has been no attempt at promoting a genuine lay spirituality and a genuine popular devotion. That is perhaps the key here because while it is true we have had movements from outside, lay movements like Marriage Encounter and the Charismatic Movement . . . one has to ask the question, Are they really suitable for our people?

'Here we are with a wonderful tradition going back to St Patrick: surely we should be able to find a very adequate and genuine popular spirituality and devotion for our people. Some would say we have to go back two hundred years to find the genuine Irish spirituality. It had a great emphasis on God's presence amongst people and in things in his creation; also a great devotion to the Scriptures, and quite a number of other things which have been lost in the last two hundred years. We must drink from our own wells. We have a wonderful well of spirituality in the Irish context.'

I went to one of the other sites where a Madonna was said to move. This time the grotto was in a wooded glade. It was daylight, and while many hundreds of people came and went in the two hours I was there no one I spoke to witnessed anything untoward. Earlier, however, some children had claimed that the statue had spoken to them and, I was told, they had relayed the messages to the crowd.

In many ways it was a bizarre weekend. In almost any other part of the British Isles the events I was reporting on would have been dismissed as so improbable as to be of little concern. Anyone seeing a moving statue would have been labelled mad. But here in Ireland dozens of friendly, rational and intelligent people talked of the improbable events they had witnessed or heard about in a totally matter-of-fact manner.

Madonna Mania however is now part of history. Not long after my visit the crowds began to drift away and at Ballinspittle the whole episode came to an abrupt end when some Protestant fanatics smashed the statue.

The people of the area no doubt still look back on the events of the summer and autumn of 1985 as the miracle of Ballinspittle, but to me the true miracle was that I had successfully taken on a demanding assignment and completed it to my satisfaction and that of the BBC, within a short time of having been in hospital suffering from severe renal failure.

My trip to Ireland was in many ways the key turning point. From that moment on I knew what my health would now allow me to do. I knew the limitations of being on dialysis but also the opportunities the treatment offered to me to lead a full, active life. I began to look forward again to the things I could hope to achieve. Far from being the end of my useful life, as I had feared, my time on dialysis has been one of the most creative professionally.

5
MOVING FORWARD

We have now lived in our present house in Kent for over three years. Dialysis has become a routine and thankfully I have suffered no complications and have not needed to return to East Ward as an in-patient. One of the results of dialysis has been that I have seen more of the family in the last three years than I did in the three years before.

However, the children are now mostly away. David is now a student of mechanical engineering at Brighton. Caroline has started working at a large hotel in Canterbury and hopes to go into hotel management. Helen and I have become 'JUNKIES', Just Us No Kids. Helen is working for the University of Kent as information officer, having spent three very successful years with Kent County Council. We have a small house in a quiet and pleasant setting. It is in a hamlet by a creek and is reached along a winding lane past orchards and hop gardens. We own one of a terrace of new houses overlooking the houseboats in the creek. We are within walking distance of the coast and a huge overgrown disused brickyard which is now an unofficial nature reserve.

The parish is served by a medieval church that is separated

from the village and stands in the middle of fields. The congregation is small and I particularly like to go to the old Prayer Book services for the sense of continuity and history. During the Lambeth Conference of bishops from the worldwide Anglican Communion held in Canterbury in 1988 I invited a friend, the Bishop of Colorado, to come and take a service. He was astonished when I showed him the old door to the church and the bullet holes which are still to be found in the woodwork. 'Relics,' I told him, 'of the war. The Civil War.'

For over a year we had no minister. We now have a vicar, or more precisely a priest, whom we share with three other parishes. Geoffrey sees potential for new life and growth in the parish and I am sure we are about to see a modest revival of parish life, but I hope at the same time we do not forfeit our sense of history.

I mention these local concerns and family matters only to show how normal life can be on dialysis. I know I am fortunate enough to have had a specially demanding, exciting and rewarding career. Many people treasure the ordinary things in life and would feel alarmed if the settled pattern of their life was threatened with disruption. Once over the initial hurdle of end-stage renal failure life can be shaped again, albeit with certain restrictions. Someone wanting to live a quiet life can opt for a quiet life; someone else wishing to return to an active career can do just that.

I continued to work for BBC Radio, for a while as a reporter on 'The World at One' and as co-presenter of the Radio 4 'Sunday' programme. After two years I released myself from 'The World at One' commitment as I was starting to overstretch myself physically.

As co-presenter of 'Sunday' I worked most weekends. I would arrive at Broadcasting House in London at about six on Saturday evening and work until eleven or twelve o'clock. There would be the script to write and some interviews to be recorded and I would generally be contributing ideas to shape the programme. Then after a brief night's sleep it was up at six to return to the studio for the transmission. Normally my co-presenter Clive Jacobs was responsible for making sure we were finished on time and did not over-shoot the Greenwich time signal before the news at eight o'clock. I usually had one or two major interviews to conduct live. I enjoy live broadcasting, even early in the morning. The programme must have a very high proportion of horizontal listeners—many people tell me they hear it in bed—but I do not think of the three quarters of a million people tuning in. I imagine I am speaking to one or two people and sometimes I am concentrating on the interview in hand so much that I forget there are thousands of other people listening. Nevertheless before each broadcast, at twenty to eight, I always felt a few butterflies in the tummy before we got into our stride.

Shortly after getting in to the swing of work again I was also asked if I would join the team of reporters working on the ITV network film documentary series, 'The Human Factor'. The programme is produced by Television South and the invitation came from Peter Williams who is in charge of factual programmes and with whom I have worked many times in the past. He and Andrew Barr, the head of religious programmes at TVS, were very accommodating, knowing the restrictions on my time dictated by the kidney machine, and in all I was involved in eighteen programmes plus a Channel 4 series on the Lambeth Conference and a programme about the Channel Tunnel.

My work for TVS took me to many parts of Britain, to America, Ireland and France. For one programme I joined a film crew in New York to meet a remarkable woman living in Harlem called Mother Hale and to tell her story. She looked after abandoned babies, often the children of drug abusers. Sometimes the children themselves were damaged by the drugs. It was a rough part of town but Mother Hale, who was well over seventy, was, just by her example, an extraordinary influence on the area. Mothers who were addicts and who often had criminal records held her in great respect. The police, too, held her in high esteem as she and her daughter, who was a doctor, went about their work.

On another trip to America I joined the former president Jimmy Carter at a work camp in Atlanta, building homes for the homeless. He was dressed and was working as a carpenter putting up a home for a young black couple. We talked to him and the former first lady about the work and the contrast between it and being in the White House. He struck me as a very good man. But, if the election result of 1980 is to be believed, he was not a good politician. Perhaps good and honest people never are.

Keeping to the diet in foreign places can be tricky, so before setting out for Atlanta I telephoned British Airways to ask if they could provide special food for me during the flight. Yes, they said, that was part of the service. I proceeded to tell them of my requirements; low protein, low potassium, low salt.

When the food arrived it was marked correctly and the low salt and low protein requirements had been met. However, the potassium content of the food was, to me, potentially lethal. I was offered fresh fruit such as melon and grapes in abundance. I raised the point with the cabin staff. They apologized, and by raiding the first-class cuisine we were able to concoct a suitable meal.

In Atlanta I told the British Airways office of the mistake. I was assured it would be corrected in time for my flight home. But the food served to me on the return journey was no better.

Back in England I set about complaining and even spoke to the catering manager. Next time I flew British Airways I was told there would be no problem. However, on a flight back from Boston not long ago I was given high potassium food yet again, having ordered my special diet. I raised the matter at the highest level. My researches seem to indicate that somewhere there has been a breakdown in communication between the dietician consulted and the catering staff. I have now been reassured that the problem will not happen again. I look forward to my next flight with British Airways with interest.

Some airlines, while offering certain types of medical diet, do not cater for renal patients. I was told by PanAm, for instance, that the low potassium, low protein, low salt diet was not one on their list. However, when I came to cross the Atlantic on one of their flights they had produced a special meal and it was ideal.

On two occasions I was asked to make films about people who followed special diets of their own for reasons of conscience or faith. One such film looked at religious diets from the point of view of a Muslim and a Jewish family. At one stage I had to sit in a hamburger bar while introducing the subject. I had to push aside the hamburger, tomato sauce and giant milkshake to make the point that while these were foods I could not eat for reasons of health there were some people who would reject them as an unholy combination and treat them as forbidden foods.

Earlier I had been the reporter on a film about a Buddhist monk. He was a former American helicopter pilot who had fought in Vietnam but who was now the abbot of a small monastery. His dietary regime was very severe. He and his fellow monks could only eat before noon. They were not allowed to cook and prepare food, and anything they ate had to be freely given to them by lay followers. All the food offered was placed in a bowl and they ate it with their hands as they sat cross-legged. The meal was preceded by chanting and prayer and was seen as a form of meditation. My diet appeared very lax in comparison.

Of all the people I met in the course of making the 'Human Factor' films, the most humbling was Mother Teresa of Calcutta. She was on a visit to London when I met her. She was in Britain to see her nuns and their work amongst London's homeless and unloved. She is a small, frail woman who clasped her rosary beads as we talked. We talked at one stage of illness and suffering and she told me of how she tried to give suffering a purpose. Each of her nuns is twinned with a suffering co-worker, someone who is housebound and often in pain but who has the chance to offer their suffering in prayer to support the work of her spiritual partner. It is an idea I find hard to understand. I met one of the suffering co-workers who felt a deep commitment to her prayer life. It was clear from our conversation that her association with one of Mother Teresa's nuns gave her a purpose in life.

I do not, however, have a contemplative nature. I prefer to be doing things and I think would find it very hard to turn my illness into prayer in quite that way. But suffering and redemption through suffering is a very Christian idea, though I find it one of the hardest to grasp.

The reason I find it hard to grasp is perhaps that I do not think of myself as suffering. My kidney problem is an inconvenience not a burden. I refuse to let it dominate. The time when I was really ill I did not recognize the fact. Only on looking back at the experience do I realize the truth.

In September 1988 I was appointed the BBC Religious Affairs correspondent. After working for the BBC as a freelance reporter or on short-term contracts, I was a member of staff for the first time. Before my appointment was confirmed I was asked to undergo a medical. The BBC doctor knew my medical history and had to decide how much of a medical liability I might be to the corporation. It was accepted that I would need to dialyse twice a week and would have to arrange my work around it.

I take it as a tribute to the medical staff at Canterbury and Keycol and to Michael Goggin that I was not only declared fit to take up my new post but that the BBC doctor was surprised to find just how fit I was. Many kidney patients do not work because employers do not understand kidney failure and assume that all kidney patients are hopeless invalids. I have even heard it quoted that only 13 per cent of all kidney patients are in employment. If this is the case it is a scandal.

Part of the problem, however, must be the image projected by the patients themselves. In order to raise money for kidney research and other kidney charities or to raise awareness of the need for donor organs, patients have to be presented as sick. Over the years many patients develop a pale, yellow complexion and this reinforces the image that kidney patients are in some way different. One feels for a child struck down by kidney failure whose early life is restricted by the treatment and the technology, but an adult will only really be incapacitated by the illness at the acute stage. Once back into the routine of work and family life, he or she can cope with life very well. Yet this is not widely understood and often families can become too protective and employers too wary and the adult patient is not allowed to resume a normal life. The result of this can sometimes be depression, a feeling of hopelessness and a consequent physical decline or indefinite dependence on the system.

One of the consequences of this can be financial anxiety. Without work the patient becomes dependent on the state and benefits are notoriously ungenerous. Almost all renal units have a social worker who will know his or her way through the benefits maze and it might even be worth those in employment to check if they are entitled to the benefits.

One doctor I spoke to referred to the 'professional kidney patient's syndrome'. This occurs to the patient with no other interests but the illness, who becomes obsessed with his or her misfortune in life.

Some patients are pushed into this role by the system and the inability to find work. Curiously, patients like this are often those who find it hardest to keep to the fluid and dietary restrictions. Their minds are seldom distracted from their problems and so they are particularly susceptible to the temptations of thirst and cravings for unwise food.

Perhaps I am being too harsh. Although I have felt low at times and angry and generally fed-up with the restrictions of renal failure, I am not of the temperament to let such thoughts linger and take over. That is my good fortune. If I had been made differently perhaps I too might have become a professional kidney patient. But most patients have the choice. Nearly four years ago I could have opted for the quiet life and decided to lower my horizons and shelve my ambitions. It was in my nature not to succumb. I decided to be the master of my illness, not its obedient servant. As a result, life has continued to provide interest and opportunity.

Early on I was told that I might have a transplant within a year. In saying this Michael Goggin was being uncharacteristically optimistic. I am on the transplant list and any time of the day or night I might get a telephone call to say a kidney has become available. I decided very early on that there was no point in sitting by the phone waiting for it to ring. I let the unit know where I can be contacted in an emergency but have planned life without considering the possibility that one day I might receive a new kidney. I have seen many fellow patients called, but as yet I have got nowhere near the much-coveted new lease of life. Once we had a call after midnight and I ran downstairs to answer it only to discover it was one of Caroline's boyfriends, a little the worse for drink! On another occasion Michael Goggin phoned in the evening, but only because of a problem with a muddled blood result. Each time I must admit my hopes were momentarily raised.

I now have a new definition for a transplant: it is something which happens to other people.

However, the call may come yet, and just in case I have made a point of discovering as much as possible about the procedure and the ethics involved.

6

TELLING MY STORY

In the summer of 1986 I started work on a Radio 4 half-hour documentary on the subject of kidney failure. The producer was Marlene Pease, with whom I had worked before, whose speciality is making programmes of a medical nature with lay appeal. I talked to a cross-section of renal professionals and recorded the final version of the documentary in August.

The programme, which I called 'My Machine and I', was inevitably a personal account of kidney failure but it widened out to explore other forms of treatment than haemodialysis, including transplantation. It was well publicized. A few weeks before transmission a photographer from the *Radio Times* turned up at Keycol and managed to take a picture of me on the machine, which duly appeared.

What follows is the complete transcript of the programme. It begins with my introduction to the subject.

There's nothing quite so boring as listening to other people going on about their ailments. But I'm not going to apologize for the next half-hour, even though I will be going on a bit about my kidneys and how they failed and how I now have to stick needles into my arm twice a week to dialyse and how I hope one day to have a transplant. The thing is, becoming a kidney patient gives one a view of the medical profession and the health service, its undoubted achievements, idiosyncracies, weaknesses, politics and strengths denied to most casual or occasional customers of the National Health Service.

Now, if one has to be ill, there's a lot to be said for choosing kidney failure over and above a lot of other nasty and potentially lethal diseases. To begin with medical science has for the last twenty or so years been able to keep a body going without kidneys for a good long time. Secondly, there's no stigma attached to kidney failure in the way that to admit to liver or heart failure implies one is suffering for a life of over-indulgence. And thirdly, kidney failure, at least in my case, is not a painful complaint, even though it can be very unpleasant and is certainly not recommended.

But before I launch into my own saga, what exactly are the kidneys and what do they do? All I knew before I was forced into taking a special interest was that there were two of them positioned somewhere in the middle of the back. So I asked Dr Michael Goggin at the renal unit at the Kent and Canterbury Hospital, who's been monitoring my health for the last six years, to give me a basic guide to kidney function.

'It's concerned with the excreation of salts and water, it's concerned with the excretion of the breakdown products of, mainly, protein. It helps to make red blood cells mature, so it tends to prevent anaemia. It also has a role to play in the maintenance of blood pressure, not only through salt and water balance but also through something we call the renin angiotensin system, which I won't elaborate on. It also has a role in the maturation, shall we call it, of Vitamin D. Renal patients don't necessarily absorb calcium very well—they are insensitive to Vitamin D. So absence of proper kidney function can lead to abnormalities of bone.'

So what is it that makes kidneys go wrong? Dr Goggin:

'The pathological classification is that it can be involved, be it silently, in an inflammatory process, so that in the tissue of the kidney itself gets laid down, say, antigen and antibody complexes fighting each other. That sets up an inflammation which follows in the destruction of the glomeruli, which are the filtering units of the kidney, and that eventually can lead to a sufficient loss of glomeruli to produce functional impairment of the kidney.'

Sometimes the kidneys suffer from pressure due to various blockages and there are also different types of hereditary disease. How long though can someone live without kidneys? Dr Goggin:

'The answer is somewhere between seven and fourteen days.'

What would happen to you over that period of time if you weren't treating it at all?

'You would become progressively drowsy and breathless. Your blood would become so acid that it would effect your breathing. There would be rapid breathing of a noisy variety and those would be the major symptoms.'

Which form did I have: which of the various forms of kidney failure caused my kidneys to pack up?

'In your case you got an immunoglobulin, which we call IgA, which is immunoglobulin A, deposited in your kidney and this set up your inflammation.'

I had picked up a nasty North African bug, bad sickness and diarrhoea, and suddenly found myself producing a pee rose. To begin with there was no way of telling if the blood in the urine heralded a long-term decline of kidney function or was merely a transitory phenomenon. It was not until I had a renal biopsy that the real nature of the illness was confirmed. I was stabbed in the back by a nasty-looking instrument and a sample of kidney was taken for analysis. Michael Goggin:

'This is the real way of making the diagnosis. The blood

can give you an indication that this may be the diagnosis in 50 per cent of cases. You really need to know if there are any other changes in the kidney as well. Quite often it is the development of high blood pressure that accelerates the disease, but even if you control the blood pressure it's a vicious circle: if you have high blood pressure the disease gets worse quickly, and if the disease gets worse quickly you have high blood pressure.'

That's what happened to me. Suddenly it shot up, from what I remember.

'Exactly. Yes, you followed exactly the pattern one would expect if you were progressive.'

And that was the time, I remember it very well because it was my birthday, that I came to see you and you said from now onwards you are on a very restricted diet.

'Yes, this is in an attempt to get the best out of what poor kidney you have. Once you lose about a half to a third of the functioning mass of your kidney then you come into something we call hyperfiltration, and this pressure to filter clogs up the glomeruli. It becomes progressive. You had, say, a third of kidney function then and, because it is hyperfiltering, it rapidly goes on so there is less and less and less. The introduction of a restricted protein diet does slow down the rate at which hyperfiltration will effect the kidney.'

You say restricted: it is very restricted, isn't it? I remember special bread without protein in it and the amount of meat, one needed a microscope to see.

'Well yes, if you keep the protein low then the hyperfiltration will be less.'

That ultra-strict diet lasted for over a year and was only eased a little once I had started to dialyse.

Kidney dialysis is a strange business. I had been prepared for it by having an operation on my arm, a vein and an artery were joined so that the vein would widen and strengthen in order to take the hollow dialysis needles. One curious effect was that it made my arm sound like a washing machine.

Dialysis is based on the principle of osmosis: blood is circulated from the arm through a dialyser and back into the arm again, and in the dialyser it is taken past a semi-pern.eable membrane. The other side of the membrane is the dialysate solution. And as the blood passes by the solution all the nasties in it filter through the membrane: the nasties being the poisons which the kidneys normally dispose of, which were making me drowsy, twitchy, itchy and feeling like death.

The first day on the dialysis ward is a confusing and terrifying experience. The place seemed to be full of machines making odd noises, highly-complicated equipment and blood everywhere. At Canterbury Daphne Tulloch is the sister in charge.

'I don't like to think it's like that, Tcd. Not blood everywhere, I hope.'

Well, in tubes anyway.

'Blood contained in tubes, yes. I do agree that when patients first arrive it must look very alarming, but the reassuring thing, I hope, for them is that they see eight or ten normal-looking people who appear to be able to talk and smile and chat perfectly normally who are attached to this alarming array of machines. That of course makes them realize it is perfectly possible to cope with it, this dialysis thing. And once they are over the first dialysis, which because it is strange is a bit of a hurdle, all starts to fall into place as being something it is quite possible to cope with.'

The second time round you insisted I start putting my own needles in.

'Yes, that's what is known as catching them when they are young and innocent, before they have had any chance to build up any barriers. It isn't a difficult procedure really, putting needles into your arm. We know that from years of experience; but the patients doing it themselves obviously think, (*a*) it's unpleasant and (*b*) I am not going to be able to do it and I don't really want to anyway.'

The machine itself looks incredibly complicated on first sight and bit by bit you encourage the patient to put bits of it together and understand how it works. How long does it normally take for a patient to get the hang of it?

'Some people take to it much quicker than others or are more interested in finding out or are less put off by the complex look of it. But on average about three months to be really at home with it and not be fazed when odd things go wrong.'

A certain amount of bullying I remember, to get me to remember which bit goes where.

'What we do is try to allocate one member of staff to one patient who follows that patient through from starting to train to finishing the training—in other words getting them onto home dialysis. The continuity of that helps. But you do have to push people because it's easy to fall into "Oh well, I don't really want to know about this, let someone else do it."'

What are the things that can go wrong while one is sitting on the machine?

'The more common ones are the patient's blood pressure dropping quite markedly and rapidly sometimes, which can in fact make the patient pass out, but usually makes the patient feel unwell: they vomit and have a headache perhaps, that sort of thing; needle problems, either the needle is coming adrift or getting into such a position where instead of the blood passing straight into the vein it actually leaks into the tissue causing a nasty, painful bruise; and I think probably the most dangerous one of all is blood leaking out of the system inadvertantly, some bit coming apart where you have got to work quickly so that the patient doesn't lose blood and air doesn't get into the system.'

In a place like a dialysis ward very strict rules have to be applied to prevent the spread of hepatitis and, more recently, Aids.

Eventually most patients are ready for home dialysis or are

found a place at a minimal-care unit. Both systems are cheaper to operate than haemodialysis in hospital and Britain has more patients dialysing at home than any other comparable European country. In my case I have got a place at a minimal-care unit. Four of us dialyse with the help of two assistants in a wooden building in the grounds of a hospital in Sittingbourne.

But keeping well on dialysis also involves keeping to a strict diet and taking tablets as prescribed for blood pressure, as a vitamin supplement and to bind the phosphates in the diet. Daphne Tulloch:

'To be fit on dialysis you have not only got to dialyse well and regularly but you have also got to stick to your renal diet and your fluid allowance. It's not easy—specially the fluid allowance—but of prime importance if you are going to be fit. And of course tablets which are prescribed have to be taken.'

And the fluid allowance is a litre or less in many cases isn't it?

'Yes, some people have to manage on 500 millilitres, but I think the majority of people have to manage on about 800 millilitres a day, which is very little.'

And the thing to watch out for with the food is the potassium, as the first big enemy.

'That is the most easy to explain to patients the dangers of, because if your potassium gets too high your heart stops and that's it. I think that is the most dramatic one, but what patients fail to realize or conveniently forget is that if they overstep the mark on their diet in a small way over a long period, they will be unwell.'

The potassium restriction is one of the hardest. Forbidden foods include bananas, tomatoes, mushrooms, chocolate, coffee, etcetera, etcetera, etcetera.

Haemodialysis is not, of course, the only treatment available. In recent years peritoneal dialysis has become more widely used. A patient has a tube placed in the tummy and fills the body cavity with a dialysing solution, filling and emptying every six hours or so if on the mobile system called CAPD, continuous ambulatory peritoneal dialysis. It is not a system I fancied, though many renal patients cope with it very well. Which method, however, is the most successful? I asked Dr Anthony Wing of St Thomas's Hospital in London who keeps the European statistics on all matters relating to renal medicine.

'For patients who have problems with their needles, haemodialysis could be a series of unending problems, getting connected up to the machine, but for others it could be very straightforward. For patients who get a lot of peritonitis CAPD will be painfully interrupted by nasty, serious illnesses of peritonitis, but many patients manage for year after year without any peritoneal infections. Increasingly we are getting better at CAPD and many of our patients choose it. But I would hesitate to say it is absolutely on a par with haemodialysis yet.'

For many people in Britain, however, to choose which type of treatment they want is a luxury. Many patients are not treated at all and die. Dr Wing showed me a revealing set of graphs.

If one is a patient in Britain over the age of forty-five, one has a rapidly-declining chance of being treated for kidney failure. For instance, while in France, West Germany and Italy over 120 new male patients per million of population over the age of sixty-five are accepted for treatment every year, in Britain the number is barely ten. Why, Dr Wing?

'That must be because we are selecting out the patients of the older age groups. It could be that the kidney specialists were refusing to treat older patients. In fact that is probably not true. If you go and talk to them they will tell you they are not sending people away from their renal units. It could on the other hand be that other doctors were not referring to the specialists all those patients who might benefit from treatment. We think that is what is happening and we have a certain amount of evidence on that from a survey which we conducted amongst our colleagues, general practitioners and other hospital doctors in this country. Although the general practitioners probably regard the work that I do as almost experimental, high-tech, and are a little reluctant to send their patients direct to me, I think that in practice they will seldom have to take that decision themselves, because the diagnosis depends on making blood tests and hospital investigations and therefore it will usually occur after the patient has been referred to a hospital specialist in some district general hospital.'

But a hospital presumably where there is no specialist renal unit?

'That is unfortunately likely to be the case because we have only one unit per million of population in this country on average compared to four or five per million in other comparable western European countries. There is a four-out-of-five chance that a patient referred to their local hospital will arrive in a hospital without a specialist who knows about kidney diseases and their up-to-date treatment.'

There is a British Kidney Patients Association, run by a formidable and energetic lady, Elizabeth Ward, whose son developed kidney failure while still at school. She says that hundreds of patients a year are turned down for treatment for social not medical reasons.

'There is selection of course being carried out because of a shortage of funding and because of the shortage of actual facilities; not enough renal units—we only have sixty-nine in this country and six transplant teams operating covering the whole of the UK. Therefore there has to be selection. And they are simply selected out of treatment because of social reasons. Maybe the particular unit which is looking at this patient says that they have to have home dialysis and they haven't got a suitable home. Or they haven't got a suitable partner to look after them in the home. Or perhaps they are somebody from overseas like, perhaps, an Indian or Pakistani and they have language problems. Perhaps they are not very clean sort of people—they come from poor social backgrounds and therefore they are selected out from treatment for that reason. Perhaps their IQ isn't as good as it might be, which is another reason. They haven't the slightest idea that the reason they are being selected out of treatment and are going to die is not because treatment is not known but because no treatment is made available for them. And so they have no chance of life.'

Is it purely and simply shortage of money?

'It is the shortage of money and the lack of will. Certainly there is not enough money in the health service for everything, we all know that. And certainly the renal replacement programme is a very costly programme per patient. But for heaven's sake, if the Health Service can't give priority to life, what are they thinking of? And not only life but a good quality of life as well. There are many dialysis patients who lead full and useful lives, who can walk tall and pull their weight in the community and who hold down good jobs, and there is no earthly reason why they should be selected out of treatment. They have a right to treatment.'

Dr Wing points out that every time a hospital doctor decides a patient is suitable for dialysis treatment he is committing the National Health Service to, on average, expenditure of £100,000. Despite this he says younger patients with uncomplicated renal failure are normally recommeneded for treatment.

'The straightforward patient with just kidney disease and nothing else much the matter with them will probably get through the system very quickly because there won't be any difficulty. Everybody will see very clearly that that patient should be treated. Even if it means travelling fifty miles to the local specialist centre and repeating that journey perhaps three times a week for that treatment in subsequent months, no one will hesitate to make that sort of referral. But if it is an older patient and he or she already has some heart disease or some other problems, then people may think that all this adds up to too much of an imposition and there will be less keenness to send the patient on to the specialist.'

Fortunately I was a straightforward patient: under forty, married with children, working, no other medical complications and articulate. Even so, just as I was in hospital waiting to dialyse for the first time my consultant Dr Michael Goggin was involved in a battle for resources.

'That is an on-going exercise. Obviously people who ration the money like to be able to plan how much they are going to spend. Obviously there is a finite amount of money available in the world at the moment for health care and so sometimes resources become a heartache in the management of patients with chronic renal failure.'

The cheapest form of treatment for a patient with kidney failure, and the most desirable medically, is without doubt the transplant. A patient can be given a kidney by a live donor, a relative, or be given a cadaver kidney taken from, perhaps, the victim of a road accident. The names of nearly 3,500 potential recipients are kept on a computer in Bristol. Mick Bewick is a transplant surgeon based at Dulwich in London who also operates in Canterbury and various other centres in the south-east. I asked him what happens when a potential donor is identified.

'A member of the nursing or medical staff associated with the intensive care unit where the patient is will ring up their local transplant unit and ask whether this patient is a suitable donor. The relatives will then be contacted and their permission asked; the coroner has to be asked in many instances and, if everything is yes and brain death is confirmed, then we will go and remove the kidneys in the hospital at a time convenient to the hospital and their other arrangements.'

You talk about brain death: now how is this determined?

'Basically it is the situation where your brain is so badly damaged that it will never recover. And although your heart is still going—your kidneys are still working, your liver is still working, your blood is still going round—your brain has gone. People who have got brain death, even if you use everything that you have got medically—all the life support machines and everything—and keep them going, then, despite all science can do, their heart stops and their body begins to rot in real terms, within a few days anyway.'

I have to admit it is not a nice thought that my life might be saved or enriched following someone's death, and it was a great comfort to me the other day when the widow of a former colleague of mine wrote to me saying how keen she had been that her husband's kidneys be used following the fatal road accident in which he'd been involved and how sad she had been when it had not been possible.

But let us say two kidneys are available. How does the surgeon choose which patient should benefit? Some doctors believe that a patient's tissue should be beneficially matched with that of the donor. The Bristol Centre certainly believes in that principle. Mick Bewick however is not convinced.

'We in the south-east of England are not too impressed by tissue typing or tissue matching especially with the new immunosuppressive techniques and so we would look for blood-group-compatible recipients. Then we do a test between the donor blood and the recipient blood, just the same test as is done when you are having a blood transfusion. If that test is negative, then we have maybe five or six patients all of whom will be suitable for one of these two kidneys, and then you tend to decide on medical grounds of priority: people who have been waiting longest, people who are iller and need one quicker, people who are blocking hospital beds rather than home dialysis units—which always upsets the home dialysis patients: they are always very fit and well, but they are not getting first offer. It is the patient who is actually blocking the bed in the unit who gets first offer. The tragedy is there are not enough kidneys by a long, long chalk and there are people I have seen who have not been taken on because kidneys were not available and that, in a sense, I take as a personal criticism. I have got to find the kidneys to put into these people, especially when I know there are, even today, people dying who could give their kidneys. Death is a tragedy. Death without donating their kidneys is a double tragedy because there was something useful there which that patient, that donor, could have given back to society.'

At Canterbury, however, tissue typing is considered important. What happens in practice is that Dulwich has many more transplants than Canterbury. But with modern anti-rejection drugs like Cyclosporin, how do results compare? I asked Terry Ray at Bristol if beneficially-matched kidneys had a better success rate.

'On our data base there is a clear improvement of 15 per cent taking beneficially-matched kidneys. That is in centres using only a small amount of Cyclosporin. If you turn to the centres that use Cyclosporin for most of their patients, then again we can still see a 15 per cent increase in graft survival due to matching and this is overlaid on a 10 per cent improvement due to the use of Cyclosporin. So Cyclosporin and matching are additive factors in graft survival.'

And that survival rate is well over 80 per cent after two years. In theory, local transplant surgeons are expected to offer Bristol one kidney for every one they keep for a local patient. As Mick Riggulsford explained to me when he showed me round the tissue-typing laboratory and computer centre at Bristol.

'Obviously the local surgeon wants the kidney to go into the best-matched person, but on the other hand he has got the pressure of perhaps fifty patients waiting locally for kidneys. So, weighing all things up, he keeps one and puts it into the best patient he can and he will give one to the country.'

But does the system work quite as well as that? Because it

would seem you handle only 30 per cent rather than 50 per cent of all kidneys that are available.

'Well, the system would work perfectly well if there were enough kidneys, but it is the number of kidneys that are available that is limiting transplantation. We are getting something like 1,500 or 1,600 kidneys a year and there are 3,500 people waiting. That's over two years as a waiting list. Some patients may be waiting six or seven years if they have a rare tissue type before a suitable kidney comes up for them. So the answer is let's get more kidneys. There are probably 4,000 people a year dying on life support machines, that is 8,000 possible kidneys, and if the medical profession was identifying those people as donors, or if their families were coming forward and saying, "Look, are there any organs you can use, please, because it would help us," then we could completely solve the problem.'

Another solution, says Mick Bewick, would be to transplant kidneys from other species.

'Physiologically our kidneys—human kidneys—and pig kidneys work very, very similarly. Anatomically they are very similar and size-wise they are much the same. Now the problem is, that if you put the kidney from one animal into another animal, species to species, that kidney goes black within minutes. There are newer techniques which are coming along which are probably going to make it a practical proposition within the next five to ten years.'

Renal medicine is, of course, a strange branch of medicine. For one thing, doctors and nurses who specialize in kidneys see the same patients week in, week out, and when a patient dies the sense of failure is acute.

I asked Dr Goggin if he felt that in renal medicine staff formed particularly close relationships with those in their care.

'Yes we do: they become almost part of our family: they certainly become very close friends of ours. We often get involved in the weddings in their families and the christenings, and a great dependence develops between the patient and the unit staff.'

I have tended to find in my own experience that I have become far more interested in the medical pros and cons and decisions and the balance of probabilities and even the politics of the business as well. Am I therefore a bit of a nuisance or do you encourage that approach?

'We encourage it. Obviously the discussion can go so far that it becomes something of a hindrance in the management of the patient, but most people don't let it go that far. It is important that there remains a flicker of paternalism in medicine.'

I had never really been ill before and it comes as something of a shock now to be so restricted in my lifestyle. I want to know why I am ill, and that is a question no doctor can answer, I have to search inside myself for clues. I have to come to terms with being dependent and costing society so much money to keep me alive. Why am I worth it when so many people in the world are starving? And yet I have an insatiable appetite for life, and a determination to keep living and working. And I have my family and the renal team at Canterbury and the progress of modern science to thank for making it possible for me to live something approaching a normal life. If it had not been for the progress of the last thirty years, today could have been the first anniversary of my death.

The programme, I think, went down well and I received a number of letters from listeners, many of whom were patients or related to patients. I also had some complimentary things said by my professional colleagues, which was gratifying. It was the first time, after years talking to other people and getting them to bare their inner feelings in public, that I had done anything quite so personal.

One of the letters I received was from the National Federation of Kidney Patients Associations, the alternative patients' representative body to that of Mrs Ward. I was invited to a reception they were holding in the House of Lords. Edwina Curry was there (she was then junior health minister) and I spoke to her, along with many others, about the need for a change in the law to make more transplants available. The most popular change was for the 'required request' system which operates in a number of countries abroad, whereby doctors in intensive care units are obliged to ask relatives of patients with suspected brain death whether or not they would be willing for the organs to be removed for transplantation if brain death was confirmed. Relatives can always refuse, but at the moment many relatives who would consent are not being asked. Mrs Curry did a lot of talking. I hope she did some listening as well.

More recently, I have learned that, although transplant surgeons and renal specialists favour 'required request', medical teams in intensive care units are often opposed to it. They see their primary job as saving lives, not being 'spare part' factories for the transplant teams. They fear that 'required request' may give the wrong impression to relatives and be bad for morale in their units.

The House of Lords reception was very useful as an occasion to make contacts and one person I met was Marion Stevens, whose experience in the field of renal medicine may be unique. I took her phone number and two years later, in the course of my research for this book, I contacted her and we arranged to meet.

7

FELLOW SURVIVORS

As I said at the beginning, every kidney patient's experience is unique. An individual's experience depends on three things; firstly, the type of kidney failure; secondly, the renal unit to which he or she is attached; and thirdly, his or her general outlook on life. My kidney failure gave me plenty of warning. Some cases, however, are quite unexpected and happen with great suddenness.

Marion Stevens is a doctor and her speciality is renal medicine. She is now both a renal physician, working in Middlesborough, and a renal patient. It was eight years ago that her kidneys failed dramatically during childbirth. She woke up on her own ward to find her life depending on the machinery she normally used on others. Despite her knowledge of the subject her reactions of shock, apprehension and confusion were much the same as those of any patient. As time went by she could reflect from the background of her professional training on what renal medicine could achieve, and this provided some encouragement, but she also knew first hand the limitations of the discipline.

Marion recalls little of the immediate crisis around her

own renal failure, save a faint memory of childbirth. Her son Julian was born by Caesarean section, and she remembers seeing the strange sight of her own inside reflected in the theatre mirror. She had been given an epidural anaesthetic and was conscious throughout the birth. But her next memory is one of lying in the renal unit with a shunt in her leg, dialysing. For twenty-four hours after Julian's arrival she was in a very bad way. Her face was swollen, she was passing no urine at all and her blood pressure at one point read 250/140.

She remembers with pleasure feeding baby Julian and for a while it was hoped she would recover sufficient kidney function to live a full and healthy life again. She had suffered eclampsia, which normally improves, but when she recovered from the acute stage her kidneys were irreparably damaged.

She had enormous support from the staff, her colleagues and of course her husband Geoffrey, but soon had to accept that her future lay in permanent dependence on them and medical technology. Two particular memories stay with her from her early days as a patient. Although initially she understood very little of what was going on around her because of her illness she has a very vivid picture etched in her mind which dates the events to Christmas 1981. She remembers watching pictures of the Soviet invasion of Afghanistan on the television and worrying about its possible consequences. She also recalls a more personal event; two of her medical colleagues standing at the foot of her bed as she lay hooked up to the machinery and as she lay in a position of total vulnerability, telling her it was her fault she was in her predicament and that she should have taken better care of herself when pregnant. A shouting match ensued with all three participants venting their anger to help cope with the totally-unexpected turn of events.

It is certainly not unusual for patients, their families and their friends to include anger in the gamut of emotions they feel. It does not normally last long, but it is real enough when it is there.

Marion has now been a kidney patient for ten years. In that time she has tried all three of the main categories of treatment: haemodialysis, peritoneal dialysis and transplantation. Last year she developed a mysterious, debilitating illness which lasted eight months. Despite exhaustive tests no cause was identified, though it seems unlikely that it was a by-product of her kidney failure. Recently, when I visited her and her husband at their home in the beautiful stone-built village of Carleton-in-Cleveland, she looked well and appeared very lively.

Marion has a positive attitude to life which is a very important ingredient in the successful treatment of a kidney patient. She is an active member of the local Methodist church and believes life is to be experienced to the full, keeping her renal failure in perspective as an occasional inconvenience. In that she is now on CAPD her diet and fluid intake are less strictly controlled. However, bag changes must be done regularly and according to rules of strict hygiene to avoid infection of the peritoneal fluid or peritoneum. This is most unpleasant, I am told, and can strike as a sharp abdominal pain with little warning.

CAPD, or continuous (some say chronic) ambulatory peritoneal dialysis involves the use of the peritoneum as a dialysing chamber. The peritoneum is the thin, smooth membrane lining the whole internal surface of the abdomen and the cavity it forms is filled with a special dialysate fluid and left for six hours. In that time the patient is quite free to get on with living a normal life. After six hours the 2 litres of fluid are drained out and the space refilled. In that time the undesirables in the blood usually processed in the kidneys and passed out of the body as urine pass into the dialysate fluid, and various essential minerals leach into the blood. The movement of fluid, by osmosis, also results in a net gain of fluid by the solution in the peritoneal cavity. As a result fluid is not retained in the body to cause swollen ankles and heart problems. (Osmosis is defined as the tendency, when two fluids containing differing concentrations of substances are separated by a semipermeable membrane for the substances to pass across the membrane from the higher concentration to the lower until the concentrations of both have been equalized.)

Emptying and replacing the fluid is a chore which takes up to half an hour each time. Marion showed me how it is done.

A CAPD patient has a cannula, a length of tubing about a foot long protruding through the skin from the peritoneal cavity. The cannula usually emerges from a site just below the navel and a little to the right or left. The tube is inserted in hospital under either a local or general anaesthetic. Marion recalls the insertion being marginally unpleasant. She felt she wanted to grab at it as it went in and experienced a sensation in the bottom as the tubing inside found its correct position low down in the peritoneal cavity.

A cannula varies in size according to the size of the patient and it is important that the point of entry is water-tight. Just below the skin, between the surface and the cavity, the tube is fitted with a cuff to keep it secure and to keep the fluid from leaking out.

Peritoneal dialysis has been available since the 1920s, at least in a primitive form, but the new designs of cannula have made it far more available. In the past a hollow needle was used and a new insertion was required every time treatment was given. There was no way a patient, even as recently as the 1960s and 1970s, could have the treatment and enjoy anything like the freedom a CAPD patient enjoys today. The improved system came from Canada in 1978 and was, after initial professional caution, in general use by the early 1980s.

A patient on CAPD can, between fluid exchanges, live an almost entirely unrestricted life. It is even possible to cover the external tubing with a special dressing and go swimming, although when it comes to washing patients are normally advised to take showers rather than have a bath. It is of course crucial to keep the exit site clean.

When at home Marion uses her bedroom for the fluid changeover. She has a small device like an incubator to warm the bag of fluid to blood temperature and a Y-shaped tube which she attaches, at the bottom end, to the exposed end of the cannula. She makes the attachment in a special way which avoids touching parts of the tubing which might cause problems if not kept absolutely clean. One end of the Y is attached to a bag of new fluid and the other to an empty bag for the old fluid. Then, using a simple valve in the tube, she empties the old fluid into the empty bag. This is done by gravity with the bag being held below the height of the abdomen. When the bag is full the valve is switched to let the new fluid flow into the peritoneal cavity. The bag is held above the level of the abdomen and again gravity does the work. For Marion it is a quite painless procedure, though she does report feeling slightly uncomfortably empty inside when the old fluid has drained out and the new has not yet taken its place.

Marion opted for CAPD after being on haemodialysis and having had a transplant. She has always continued to work, except when in hospital herself as a patient, even in the early days when haemodialysis required her to be on the machine for three five-hour sessions every week.

The transplant took place after nine months on dialysis. Marion was offered a kidney by her brother Ben. Her father had offered a kidney as well but it was considered that Ben's would be the more suitable. To determine that he was a suitable donor Ben first of all had to undergo a general medical examination to ensure that he was himself fully fit. Then blood samples were taken to determine blood group and tissue type. Blood pressure was also taken and urine output tested. Then came a kidney X-ray and a rather uncomfortable test involving a catheter being introduced into a blood vessel from a site near the groin and being pushed through to the kidney for a close look.

To accept or not to accept an offer of a kidney from a living relative is a decision which can only be taken by the patient involved, once the medical all-clear is given. It never occurred to Marion not to accept the offer. She and her brother, who is nineteen months younger, had always been close. 'If our roles had been reversed,' she says, 'I would have made the same offer without hesitation.'

Ben was in hospital for six days, during which, Marion recalls, he scandalized the nurses with his daring lilac lurex underpants.

The kidney, however, did not work as well as it had been hoped. Five days after the operation Marion experienced a bad episode of rejection. The kidney stopped working and for eight weeks she continued to dialyse. It was an intense time emotionally, she recalls. Many of her friends prayed for her and she received the laying on of hands. She spent a lot of time listening to tapes of charismatic music and worship.

She shared a small ward of single isolation units with Timbo Ward who was also recovering from a transplant. It is Timbo's mother, Elizabeth Ward, who has done much through the British Kidney Patients Association to campaign for the interests of kidney patients.

Eventually Marion's kidney began to work and for a year she knew the freedom a successful transplant can bring: freedom to eat, drink and travel as one wishes. But in the end the anti-rejection drugs were not sufficient to stave off rejection, and fourteen months after the transplant the kidney had finally to be removed. It was a time of great disappointment for Marion and her brother.

For the next year and a half Marion returned to her regular sessions on the kidney machine, but then decided to try peritoneal dialysis. She saw it as a system which would keep the blood biochemistry under greater control without the fluctuations in salt, potassium, creatinine and urea associated with haemodialysis. She also saw it as a system which would give her greater freedom to work and to travel. Indeed she now finds she can travel quite freely, and the new bags of fluid are delivered to her by the manufacturers wherever she might be. On the debit side she has experienced peritonitis and needs to adjust her life and dress to cope with a length of tubing emerging from her abdomen.

More recently Marion has gained a new lease of energy from taking the drug erythropoeitin which helps build up the essential red cells in the blood. Most kidney patients have anaemia, a haemoglobin of below 8 g/dl, and get tired quickly when involved in physical activity. Taking the new drug raises the haemoglobin levels. By coincidence Marion's husband Geoffrey, who is a haematologist, was involved in the pioneering work involved in developing the new treatment.

Epo does however have two potential drawbacks. Firstly, it is very expensive, and secondly, it can work so well in thickening the blood that it contributes to clotting.

A fistula that clots and becomes sluggish can cause a whole host of problems. Marion feels the drug should not be offered to every patient but kept for patients with haemoglobin levels below 7.5 g/dl in order to raise the level to that figure. This would avoid the need to give blood transfusions which, although they do boost a patient's blood and energy levels, can cause immunological problems which make it difficult to carry out a successful transplant.

However judged, Marion Stevens must be considered a successful patient. Nevertheless, like all renal patients she has had her ups and downs and even experienced a crisis or two. On one occasion her potassium level rose alarmingly and she made a dash for the hospital because she was experiencing all the symptoms of erratic and weakening heart-beat and tingling skin that occur just before the heart finally gives up.

Despite the inevitable problems she has noticed how important it is for a patient to approach treatment with the right mental attitude in order both to survive and thrive. Patients who keep working or have a positive purpose in life, other than just existing from one dialysis to the next, do best.

In Marion's case her work as a doctor, her family and her strong Christian faith have given her good reason to keep going.

When I went to see Marion she introduced me to a number of her patients who, through their positive attitude to life, have not only weathered the storms of renal failure but gone on to lead fulfilling lives.

Paul can be justifiably called one of the pioneers of renal medicine. He spent twenty-three years on dialysis. If he had been born many years earlier or suffered kidney failure earlier, he would not have survived at all. His kidneys failed when he was in New Zealand and he returned home, a very sick young man, to begin life on one of the primitive haemodialysers of the time. He had been a farmer but found, as time went by, that he could not cope as well physically with the work and so became an agricultural salesman. He has now had a successful transplant and is contemplating a new change in his life—training for the Anglican ministry.

Billy is on haemodialysis. He had been a manual worker, specializing in demolishing chimneys. Now his driving force in life is fund raising for the local renal unit. He has a particular flare for the challenge and has found his health and his whole attitude on life has changed since he found this purpose. Like many kidney patients he relies on the skill of the medical profession but has developed a certain scepticism. He tells the story of one doctor who visited him at night when he was in considerable pain. He did not recognize him as a kidney patient and thought that he might be dehydrated by an infectious disease. When he took his pulse and felt the throbbing fistula, he leapt back with shock.

FELLOW SURVIVORS

Cindy had a transplant for two years, but for her it was not a happy experience. She now suspects the anti-rejection drugs had an effect that made her depressed. She is now on an unusual form of dialysis which is a blend of the two main systems. She dialyses through the peritoneal cavity as with CAPD but does not change fluid every six hours. Instead the exchanges are done automatically at night. The system is called CCPD (Continuous Cycling Peritoneal Dialysis). It has its restrictions as well as its advantages. During the day Cindy can work normally—she is a medical secretary—but she must always be home at night. Freedom to stay away with friends is severely curtailed. She likes people not to know she is a kidney patient and her appearance gives no reason to suspect she has kidney problems. She is unmarried and remembers how one boyfriend she had did not want to know her once he discovered about her dialysis. Another boyfriend she recalls being most helpful and understanding.

Her mother tells a story from the early days which the medical profession should be shamed by. When her problem was diagnosed Cindy and her mother decided to take a holiday before the regular dialysis commitment began. They went to America and, as luck would have it, it was there that the kidneys finally failed and Cindy needed to start dialysing. On her return to Britain they encountered one nurse at a renal unit who must have been afraid no doubt of cross-infection. Cindy and her mother heard her say, 'She should be sent home to die, we don't want her here.'

Joyce works in a tax office and has dialysed for eight years, with few problems. She dialyses at a hospital unit in the evenings and remembers the early days when dialysers, which are now disposable, were reusable. It involved an hour's work to clean up after treatment. She is married and again there is no way of telling by looking at her that she is a dialysis patient. She is an example of the many kidney patients who get on with a normal life with little fuss, coping with the inconvenience of dialysis without allowing it to dominate.

Fred kept working through eight years of dialysis. He is a bricklayer and his illness did not hamper him unduly. Then came the chance of a transplant and he became only the second person in the United Kingdom to receive a kidney donated by his wife. It was discovered their blood groups and tissue types were sufficiently well matched for the operation to go ahead and Fred now has all the new energy, and the ruddy complexion, of a person with a successful transplant. The only disadvantage he has noticed is that he now gets more colds than before.

It would be a mistake to assume that all these patients have been free of troubles. Joyce reports being tired in the mornings and needing to make an extra special effort to get into work on some days. All have to cope with restrictions, and the limits on diet and fluid intake for those on haemodialysis are the most constantly demanding. What they have in common with Marion Stevens is their determination not to let the illness dominate their lives. In the early days, when the kidney failure is new and frightening and one feels particularly wretched, it is hard to realize that one day life will return. But it does, if in life one has something one wants to return to. What Paul, Billy, Fred, Joyce and Cindy all demonstrate is that kidney failure can be kept in perspective. It is an inconvenience and a nuisance but not something which in the long run should take over one's whole being.

8
FAITH AND HOPE

I first met Gail Lawther when she was the 'Sunday' programme guest one weekend in 1988. I was at the time co-presenting the programme, and every week we were joined on the air by a guest who would help us review the current religious press. It was the way the 'Sunday' programme traditionally started its fifteen minutes on the air before the weather forecast and news at 8 a.m.

Gail had been given a pile of publications, *The Church Times*, *The Methodist Recorder*, *The Catholic Herald*, *The Tablet* and many others. She is a journalist herself—was then the editor of a Christian woman's magazine—and she was asked to select items of particular interest to her.

How we got on to the subject of kidneys I do not recall, but off the air that was the topic that came up. I discovered that Gail's husband Chris and I had something in common: kidney failure. The only difference was that Chris was enjoying the benefits of a successful transplant.

A few months later we met for lunch. Sitting in the BBC's canteen we swapped notes on the subject of renal medicine and treatment and Chris told me of his experience as a patient.

Chris's kidney problems had started much earlier than mine. At the age of five he had had one of his kidneys removed following nephritis. Throughout his childhood his health was watched, but he had no special problems and it was not until he became a student that his remaining kidney started causing difficulties. He was at Reading University studying typography and graphic communication. It was in his fourth term that symptoms began to emerge which were to lead to total renal failure.

He remembers the feeling of lethargy, a loss of his usual concentration span and increased irritability. He recalls going round the National Gallery in London as part of his course and having to sit down in every gallery to recover from the effort feeling distressed and tearful. His doctors wondered if it was all due to overwork but he had blood tests taken and just after his twentieth birthday, at the end of November 1976, he was admitted to St Bartholomew's Hospital in London, where his father was a consultant.

So began a long association with Barts, the famous teaching hospital, which, despite the family connections, was not a completely happy one.

His first few days were spent on emergency peritoneal dialysis. He felt wretchedly ill and was subjected to a whole battery of tests and treatments. At one stage he had a drip in his arm, a shunt in his leg and an operation to build a fistula in his other arm. Visitors who saw him at the time remember him looking very ill because he had lost a great deal of weight.

To start with haemodialysis was a very unpleasant experience. His first half-a-dozen sessions left him feeling extremely ill and the whole business was compounded by his intense dislike, even fear, of needles.

After a month of twice-weekly dialysis his fluid retention levelled out and the time came for the fistula to be used and the shunt in his leg removed. This latter procedure Chris describes as five minutes of brutality.

The dialysis unit at Barts was away from the main hospital in a Portacabin block in the grounds of an old workhouse in London's East End. Because of his family connection with the hospital he knew some of the staff, but this connection had another side to it. As Chris's father was a consultant some of the staff found it a bit awkward and embarrassing to deal with him, and were rather brusque, although most were sympathetic.

Chris was one of the younger patients and it was in his nature to ask questions and to think about what was happening to him and about what he was told to do. In due course he returned to his studies at Reading and arrangements were made for him to dialyse at the university health centre. It was an arrangement which suited him well and he had the freedom to decide when to spend time on the machine, as long as he did the required hours every week. Perhaps because he was too independent and questioning, he sensed relations with the Barts consultant deteriorating. At one time Chris was accused of not dialysing, when in fact he had done so. 'There was one big row,' Chris recalls, and for a long while the atmosphere was tense. In the end, in 1982, Chris moved from a design job in London to become design studio manager for a company in Worthing, West Sussex, and so he transferred to a new unit, at Brighton.

By this time Chris and Gail were married. She had known him when his illness first landed him in hospital and had visited him there.

Chris was in his student days a lapsed Catholic. He had been brought up as one and had tried the church in Reading but was left unmoved. By the time he and Gail were considering marrying, Gail had become an evangelical Christian. It was an approach to religion which Chris initially found strange. He resented the idea that evangelicals thought they had got it right. But he was incredibly curious about it all and spent a lot of time thinking. He knew God was there as he saw him in creation, but exactly how God should be approached and understood was something he was not sure about. As a student he had plenty of time to ponder such matters. There was a nurse on the renal unit who was a Christian who chatted with Chris, and in June 1977 Chris decided that the evangelical approach made sense to him. He was still a bit unsure about creation and evolution, but the main tenets fitted.

Gail describes Chris as a fighter. 'If it had been me I might have given up and decided to go off to heaven. But he was determined he wasn't going to let his medical problems interfere with life.' He dialysed overnight so that work and leisure time would not be affected; he played sport and went away for holidays and weekends as often as possible.

Indeed Chris goes as far as saying that, given his life again, he would have wanted to go on dialysis, though not perhaps for so long. 'I had been lazy and ill-disciplined, God needed to bring me up with a shock. It was an amazing eye-opener. You can't afford to stray from the discipline of dialysis and diet. The effect of the experience worked off into the rest of my life. I am now much less nervous about things, more peaceful and less self-centred.'

Some partners are intimidated by the idea of coping with illness. Gail was not so threatened. With a brother who has haemophilia she was used to matters medical being constantly in the background in the family and she was intrigued by Chris's machine.

They discussed with a senior registrar at Barts if they would have any special problems as a married couple. They asked if they could have children and were reassured that they could. Chris's parents, however, were given a different story: that it was a well-known fact that kidney patients cannot have children. But believing they could be parents themselves when the time came, Gail volunteered to take part in a trial for a new contraceptive. Only later did she see the irony of that, when she realized, because of Chris's illness, she could not have children. She hopes that she and Chris did not invalidate the findings.

FAITH AND HOPE

The truth, as I understand it, is that while being a kidney patient does diminish fertility it is not impossible for a man on dialysis to father a child. For a woman, again, fertility is diminished but not totally extinguished, though many doctors will advise women against becoming pregnant in case the pregnancy produces problems which could harm the mother or child. The fertility problem is not entirely solved by transplantation as some of the immunosuppressive drugs can effect fertility. In some cases the original renal disease irrevocably damages fertility and a transplant cannot change that.

When Chris started dialysing in 1976 he was told he would have a three-year wait for a transplant. In the event he waited ten. While his time as a dialysis patient based on Brighton renal unit was far more relaxed than his time with Barts, towards the end of the ten years dialysis was becoming an increasing chore.

Chris and Gail became used to the day-by-day living all kidney patients get to know. On two or three occasions Chris had good cause to believe that he was close to death. One instance involved a portable dialysis machine. A routine ammonia test which was part of using the machine showed positive. For a while he had no idea if his blood had been affected, he just had to wait. He curled up in bed, said goodbye to Gail and 'See you in heaven'. His fears were not realized, but it was moments like that which he feels showed the reality of his new maturity and faith.

When eventually after ten years of dialysis Chris received the transplant call, he approached the possibility of a new lease of life with caution. Once before he had been summonsed and was all prepared for surgery when he reacted badly to a blood transfusion and the operation was called off. As he heard later it was a false negative and he could have had the transplant, but it was not to be. Chris recalls Gail turning as white as a sheet with the shock of the last minute let-down and even the doctors looking upset at the anticlimax. Reflecting on the dashed hopes Chris again drew on his faith. 'Perhaps God knew it was not the right time. I was doing well on dialysis and had important exams to take.'

However, as time passed and brought no news of a transplant Chris became increasingly depressed. He knew many of his friends were praying that he might have a new kidney, and yet ten years had passed since his kidney failure and he was still depending on dialysis. From time to time he would have a telephone call in the night. His hopes would be raised for a moment until he discovered the caller had dialled a wrong number. He carried a radio pager with him. It sounded from time to time and gave him new false alarms. It was a testing time for his faith. Why, he wondered, did God appear to answer small prayers but not the big one?

Eventually, in February 1987, it happened. They were told by the renal unit that a kidney might become available. Things were looking bad for a woman in the intensive care unit. Chris and Gail, who were about to set off on holiday, decided to delay leaving. Chris remained calm but went through the dilemma many patients experience. As keen as he was for a new kidney, he could hardly hope that the young woman whose life was on a knife edge should die.

His prayer the night before the operation was simply, 'Lord, if this is your time for me to have the operation then so be it.' He dialysed that evening and by the next morning had convinced himself that indeed it was better that the girl recovered and he could wait.

It was at that moment that the hospital called. The operation was to go ahead. Chris was prepared for the theatre and by the afternoon the surgeon had given Chris a new kidney.

Chris remained in hospital for nine days. For the first five he had a catheter in place to drain the urine from his bladder and his instructions were to drink, drink, drink. He needed one further bout of dialysis and it took several days before he was convinced that things were going well. It is an anxious time for all patients. As every test is taken there is the worry. Will it show the kidney working? Will there be signs of rejection?—questions which counterbalance the tremendous excitement of realizing that the future will bring new freedom without dialysis. Chris knew that many people had prayed for him over the years and felt that he had a large credit account in the Prayer Bank on which to draw.

It took him quite a few months to feel totally physically secure. He had a new scar, a lot of bruising and the constant feeling that his new kidney could be damaged if he was not careful. But very soon he noticed the benefits. The fidgets and tensions had gone and sleep was less disturbed. Sometimes the fidgets had been so bad that Gail had had to retreat to the spare room to get some sleep.

When I last saw Chris he was celebrating two years with his new kidney. Dietary and fluid restrictions had been lifted and he was in extremely good health.

His story, while special to him, is typical in many ways. Long periods of time on dialysis can lead to feelings of depression, wondering if the sentence is ever to be lifted. The false alarms waiting for a transplant are inevitable and one should never think 'this is it' until all the hurdles have been cleared. Even after the operation there is a long period of uncertainty. New kidneys can start well and then reject or take an age to get going and then survive.

Chris and Gail were sustained by their faith: a belief that God is ever present, can intervene in one's life and is in charge. It is an approach which can lead to problems, particularly if God does not appear to be answering the petitions made to him. Faith must then be maintained through thick and thin and the Christian must believe that everything will be right in God's good time and in his way.

Kidney failure can also present a Christian with other moral dilemmas. One of which is this: when to tell the truth about the kidney disease to potential employers? Chris remembers being offered a job, a much-coveted job, by a very well-known firm. When they discovered he was a kidney patient, even though his dialysis was not going to interfere with his work, they withdrew their offer. From that moment onwards Chris knew that he might have to avoid being too honest when applying for jobs. The public perception of a kidney patient as someone who is constantly in bad health and therefore a less reliable employee needs correcting. Indeed many kidney patients are so good at monitoring their health that they have fewer days off sick than normal, healthy employees.

It cannot be argued that those with a strong faith, of whatever sort, can guarantee to do better as kidney patients. Again, what can be argued perhaps is that those who think beyond their illness, who have horizons that are not limited by the treatment and the disciplines imposed by it are those who tend to do best.

In the case of Chris and Gail, they see their faith as giving them the strength to rise to every new challenge, to look beyond the apparent limitations imposed by the illness. They are both convinced they would not have coped as well without that faith.

9
QUESTIONS OF LIFE AND DEATH

In April 1989 the Canterbury Kidney Patients Association invited the transplant surgeon Geoffrey Koffman to address its annual general meeting. There was a very high turnout at the meeting and after the business section Mr Koffman spoke about the transplant programme in the south-east of England.

He acknowledged that Canterbury patients had not had a fair deal. Patients based on the London hospitals had a better chance of getting a transplant. One year, he said, Canterbury had only had two. This was partly due to the uneven supply of kidneys but also, he accepted, partly to do with the fact that the transplant surgeon was based in London. He outlined how he hoped to improve the situation and assured the audience that Canterbury patients would be treated fairly in future. He said, however, that they would probably be called to Guys' hospital in London for the operation as the expertise was all based there and having a central point for transplantation saved the surgeon having to drive up and down from London.

At question time I asked him if he had undertaken earlier that year to carry out twenty transplant operations on Canterbury patients in 1989. He said that figure was now his annual target but that in recent months the supply of kidneys had dwindled and that now he hoped to carry out fifteen. Maybe I shall be one of them.

To put it bluntly, new kidneys for transplantation come from dead people. About 20 per cent of the population has signed a kidney donor card, but not everyone carries the card all the time. Every year enough kidneys in theory become available (as a result of people dying from head injuries and similar causes which leave the kidneys healthy and functioning) for everyone on the waiting list to receive a kidney without having to wait more than a few months to a year. The problem is turning potential donors into actual donors and this involves delicate diplomacy by hospital staff in approaching relatives.

A very informative article appeared in *The Nursing Times* in 1987 on the subject written by Josephine Richards, the sister in charge of the intensive care unit at the Royal Devon and Exeter Hospital. A nurse in an intensive care unit is ideally placed to describe the way donor organs are collected, as in almost all cases donor organs come from such units. If a patient dies in a car crash and arrives at hospital with no heart beat and no sign of life it is too late to retrieve a kidney.

Josephine Richards began her article by describing the care received by a patient arriving at an intensive care (or therapy) unit, when to begin with the object of all medical attention is to make the patient comfortable and to save life. She describes the various procedures followed to monitor temperature, blood pressure, etc. After a while, however, with some patients it becomes apparent that recovery is not possible, as the patient shows little prospect of regaining consciousness and appears totally unaware of what is going on around.

To quote Josephine Richards's article:

At very close, regular intervals observation of the pupils is carried out. They will probably have been fixed and dilated since admission. If however they are reacting and of normal equal size any changes must be reported immediately to the medical staff.

When the patient has been thoroughly examined, diagnosed as far as possible, adequately assessed and settled, the next-of-kin must be interviewed. They will have already been seen by a doctor in the accident department and told that the patient is critically ill.

The interview should be carried out by the anaesthetic consultant in charge of the unit. If this is not possible, the senior registrar or registrar will see them. A nurse also attends the interview to prevent conflicting reports.

The seriousness of the problem must be emphasized from the start. The family must be made aware that the patient is severely brain damaged and that he may not survive. They are told, in very simple terms, that he is attached to a breathing machine. If he is being sedated and relaxed this too is explained as is the visual display unit and monitoring equipment. The need for a blood transfusion is also explained.

They are asked if the patient has any underlying illnesses or if he is receiving any medical treatment.

They are given the opportunity to ask questions. At this particular time questions often do not come to mind. They are assured that the nurses will answer any questions later.

A time is arranged for the next interview. They are told that should the patient deteriorate they will be informed immediately. Hospital accommodation should be offered to them so that they can be at hand.

Also at this point, or before if time has permitted, any student nurses or new staff who are not familiar with the procedures are reassured. The importance of the care of the patient and relatives is fully explained to them.

While the patient is in the unit total medical and nursing care are given. Care of the family is just as important. While he is lying in a hospital bed, looking pink, feeling warm, with a visual heart beat and his chest rising and falling, it is extremely difficult for the relatives to believe that he is going to die. A great deal of time needs to be spent talking to them. They must also be allowed to develop trust in what they have been told.

At any time after admission to the unit, the patient's condition is likely to deteriorate. If this happens, immediate steps are taken to treat any problem if he is thought to be a potential donor.

Three conditions must be met before the diagnosis of brain stem death can be considered.

If these criteria are met, the possibility of the patient's being an organ donor is considered, if there are no contraindications to the use of the organs. If there are none, blood is sent to the laboratory for tissue typing, hepatitis surface antigen, HIV, biochemical and blood glucose screening.

The first examination for brain death must be carried out either by two consultants or one consultant and one other doctor who must have been qualified for more than five years. One of the consultants will usually be the consultant in charge of the unit. Neither of the doctors must be members of the transplant team.

To record the results of the examination, we in Exeter have designed a special diagnosis of brain stem death form. The form is divided into a group of five headings. Each group of headings contains further questions. If the answer to all these questions is 'no' the patient is presumed stem dead, although a second set of tests must be done to confirm this.

At this time, the next-of-kin must be interviewed again. Ideally, they are seen by the same doctor, who is accompanied by a nurse. They will then be told the 'special test' has been performed, the findings of which suggest that brain stem death has occurred. Another full explanation of this is given to them. They will require a great deal of support.

After the first examination for brain death, contact is made with the transplant co-ordinator who is informed that an organ donor might be available. The relatives sometimes offer organs for transplantation at this time. When they realize that there is absolutely no hope for survival, they may think of how they can help others. If this happens, it is a lot easier for the staff who do not have to approach the subject directly.

There is no set time between making the brain death tests. A great deal depends on how the family react. They may find great difficulty in accepting the news. If the second test can be delayed for a while, they have more time to adapt to the situation. Equally once they realize the patient is clinically dead, they may wish the second test to be carried out fairly soon to relieve the patient of any further indignity. It can be very upsetting for the medical and nursing staff if too long is allowed between tests.

As soon as the second examination has been completed, the patient is certified dead. The form is completed and signed by both doctors.

The next-of-kin must now come to terms with the fact that the patient is, in fact, dead. He or she must understand that there is no point in continuing with mechanical ventilation. A great deal of time and patience will be required to explain this finally. It should be done in very simple terms and each factor taken separately. Time must be given to allow them to ask questions. They may ask if they have to make the decision to 'switch off the breathing machine'. They are assured that this will be done by the doctor.

Once the relatives fully understand the position, the question of organ donation can be broached. They may have already thought about it and sometimes they will have discussed it between themselves. On the other hand, the idea may fill them with complete horror. They may not have thought about it and need time for consideration. If they do need time we try to allow this. Occasionally, though, the patient's condition may be deteriorating and time may not be on our side. Each time the situation is a little different and one has to act accordingly.

If the answer to the question is a definite 'no' the subject is closed.

In the event of there being no next-of-kin available at the time of death, the health authority automatically takes possession of the body and may then authorize the removal of organs for transplantation.

After the patient has been certified dead, the relatives are encouraged to visit the patient again to say their 'goodbyes' and encouraged to go home. The heart-beating cadaver is taken to the operating theatre and the organs are removed. Mechanical ventilation is discontinued.

From the time the patient is admitted to the unit, he will require total medical and nursing care. Even if it is known the situation is hopeless this must continue.

The consultant anaesthetist gives a talk on brain stem death to student nurses and a sister or charge nurse from the unit also gives a talk on the subject of ITU. The question of 'switching off' the ventilator always comes up. At interview all trained staff are asked their views on both switching off the ventilator and transplantation.

The concept that death of the brain means that the patient is dead is often difficult to grasp, therefore, with the transplantation of more organs taking place each day and the increasing need for donors, the way relatives are approached is very important. All relatives react in different ways and need to be treated accordingly.

I have quoted the above as many patients on the transplant list think about such things and worry that their good fortune in getting an organ might cause additional stress to bereaved families. But there is a growing volume of evidence to suggest that many families of people who die in ITU are grateful that their personal tragedy can bring hope to someone else. After a transplant families like to have news of the recipient. It is standard practice, however, not to reveal to the recipient the identity of the donor, although often this information leaks out. I feel that it might help a recipient to know something about the donor. It is possible that rejection of a donated kidney could be psychological as well as biochemical and a patient needs to feel comfortable mentally and physically with the new addition to his or her body. In Newcastle the transplant co-ordinator acts as a go-between, and donor families and recipients can write to one another. Sometimes they meet — and there have been no reported complications.

I have also quoted Josephine Richards extensively to show how carefully the unit strives to keep the patient alive while there is still hope of life and to show that relatives are approached about organ donation in a sensitive manner. Exact procedures will vary from hospital to hospital but by and large the Devon and Exeter experience is typical. Some units do not produce as many organs as others and the idea of changing the law to require staff to broach the subject of organ donation has much to commend it.

From the patient's point of view the transplant is a time of apprehension and excitement. The success rate is improving. While there are some disappointments, such as grafts which fail after a few days, there are many transplant patients who have survived many years. And even if the graft fails all is not lost as the patient returns to dialysis and when conditions are right can be given a second operation.

When a surgeon has a list of patients and knows a kidney is about to become available the first task is to identify which patients are blood-group compatible. The next is to see if there is a patient with a close tissue match. If there is more than one patient to choose between the surgeon will then enquire which patients are fit to have the operation and which patient has been waiting long or is in great need.

When a patient has a transplant he or she can expect to be

in hospital for anything from ten days to three months, depending on how quickly the kidney takes. To begin with large doses of immunosuppressive drugs are given; the doses are decreased as time goes by. There will never, however, be a time when the drugs are entirely abandoned. Some of the drugs have side effects. One is to make the patient hairier. Another can lead to depression. Patients also put on weight, although that is as much to do with the diet being lifted as anything else. A few patients have reported a considerable increase in libido following a transplant: this is not a drug side effect but just the returning of a feeling of well-being.

In the early days a patient will have a catheter to the bladder but this is soon removed. After three months the patient may have an operation to remove a small tube inside.

A successful transplant is undeniably the best treatment for kidney failure. First of all it costs well over £10,000 a year to keep a patient alive on haemodialysis, whereas a successful transplant patient costs the taxpayer around £3,000 a year. From the patient's point of view a transplant gives new energy and new freedom. But a transplant operation always involves risk and a small percentage of patients do not benefit. They suffer bouts of rejection and hospitalization sometimes for no good outcome. Approximately 80 per cent of grafts are successfully working after one year and continue to work well, although rejection continues over the years. After five years about half of all grafts are likely to have rejected. But from the patient's point of view, even just five years are seldom wasted.

Some surgeons believe that within the next five or ten years the problems of rejection will have been overcome. Some even say that the supply of kidneys will be limitless as they could in future come from pigs. Pigs' kidneys are very similar in size and make-up to human kidneys. If these advances are made it will be the effective end of dialysis of all kinds.

In the meantime human kidneys are required and often the willingness of relatives to offer organs and of staff to ask is affected by the news. A few years ago a BBC television documentary questioning the diagnosis of brain death used before removing organs had a sharp impact. For many months the supply of kidneys was reduced substantially. On the other hand, when the television programme 'That's Life' highlighted the case of the little boy, Ben Hardwick, who was in desperate need of a liver transplant, the supply of organs increased. Early in 1989 there were stories in the newspapers about impoverished Turks offering their kidneys for sale. One potential donor needed money urgently to buy medical treatment for his daughter. It is now illegal to sell organs, but in recent years certain doctors have made a lot of money from this unscrupulous trade.

At the height of the controversy I was telephoned one morning by the Radio 2 'Jimmy Young Show'. I was dialysing at the time but they wanted to speak to me as a kidney patient and as the religious affairs correspondent about the ethics and morality of the trade in organs. We pulled my machine and my chair across the room and I was just able to reach the telephone and I did a live interview there and then. I was quite clear in my mind that the whole business was unsavoury and unethical. It is one thing, indeed a great act of love, for a relative to give an organ; but for someone to be forced into selling an organ through poverty or desperation seems to me wholly wrong.

It can be argued that there will always be abuses of the system as long as there is an overall shortage of legitimate kidneys for transplant. One of the reasons for this is the public reaction to the latest news about organ donation, but another reason concerns the medical profession.

Seven years ago there was a case of a family of a young man who was killed in a motor cycle accident. He was on a life support system and was an ideal potential kidney donor. He had discussed with his family before the accident the subject of organ donation and carried a donor card. The family, however, had to volunteer his organs and more than once ask a reluctant medical team to consider him as an organ donor.

The resistance to organ donation can come from the medical staff as well as relatives. ITU medical teams know that an organ donor is a disruption to routine. The equipment needed to keep the kidney in a usable state may be needed urgently to save life. Some hospitals dislike their facilities being taken up by organ transplant surgeons who come to retrieve kidneys, livers, hearts and lungs. There is also a feeling shared by many ITU staff that transplant teams take them for granted. Their primary job, they emphasize, is to save lives, not to be a human spare parts factory.

And once the kidneys are retrieved they may not be used to best effect, being put into a local patient and not given to the best tissue match. The politics and psychology of organ transplantation is complex. One obvious way to increase the supply of kidneys would be to tackle the fact that 30 per cent of all relatives approached refuse permission. Sometimes this is because they have not accepted the death; sometimes it is because they feel they do not want the body 'cut about'.

I must be one of the few potential recipients actually to have witnessed a transplant. This happened in Newcastle, when I was filming a documentary for ITV. It was a fascinating experience, and I fully agree with the surgeon who said that to see a kidney swell and come to life on the operating table inside its new owner, and to see the first dribbles of urine within seconds, is the most marvellous sight in all medicine.

10

FACING THE DIAGNOSIS

Most people start life with a pair of healthy kidneys. Each is about 10 centimetres long and they are found on either side of the spine in the middle to low part of the back. A kidney is a complex organ with a variety of essential functions. Typically a kidney contains around a million minute filters called nephrons and each nephron is served by a cluster of tiny blood vessels called a glomerulus. Good working kidneys cope with a throughput of up to 800 litres of blood a day and produce some 180 litres of filtrate. Much of the filtrate is re-absorbed as it contains fluid and minerals and protein essential to health but the remainder is excreted as urine. Average urine ouput is around 1.5 to 2 litres a day.

But the kidneys are not just a giant filtering plant. They are a regulating organ keeping such substances as glucose, protein, amino-acids, water and minerals in the right balance. They are also a manufacturing plant turning vitamin D into a hormone which keeps the bones in good shape. Very importantly the kidneys help produce red blood cells by producing erythropoetin which stimulates the production of these cells in the bone marrow. And last but not least the kidneys perform an essential role in controlling blood pressure. Thus it is that anaemia, or a shortage of red blood cells, and erratic blood pressure are common symptoms suffered by patients with ailing kidneys.

Kidneys fail in one of two basic ways. Acute renal failure is often reversible but happens normally with great speed. It can happen as a result of someone being involved in an accident which damages the kidneys or as a result of a blockage in the urinary system causing back pressure to build up. Acute failure might also be precipitated by a patient's reaction to a drug or from a drop in blood pressure.

Chronic renal failure is by definition irreversible and normally builds up over a long period of time. It can be caused by a variety of factors including high blood pressure, a kidney infection, diabetes or by an inherited condition.

Because a person can survive very healthily with only one kidney, and indeed with only part of one kidney operating correctly, there is enough renal capacity left for the body to be able to cope even when renal failure has reached an advanced stage. Consequently a person can have diseased kidneys in steady decline and not be aware of the problem. Only if there is some reason for a blood or urine test to be made— perhaps if blood has been noticed in the urine or in the course of a routine medical examination — does the problem come to light. And after the tests on blood and urine samples and a monitoring of blood pressure it is often not until a renal biopsy is taken that the exact nature of the renal failure emerges.

A renal biopsy involves a small sample piece of kidney being removed and examined in the laboratory. It is an uncomfortable process and done with the patient being conscious and, ideally, co-operative. It takes the form of an unpleasant stab in the back with a special probe. I would recommend anyone about to undergo such a procedure to ask the doctor how many renal biopsies he or she has previously done. It is not wise to be a nervous medic's first subject!

FACING THE DIAGNOSIS

When what is known as end-stage renal failure approaches, dialysis treatment is required and a variety of symptoms emerge. Uraemia occurs when 80 to 90 per cent of kidney function has been lost. This condition is literally urine in the blood. To begin with a patient feels off colour; then, as time passes, the feeling grows more persistent and the sufferer feels itchy. Headaches and vomiting are often signs, especially with a rise in blood pressure. As renal failure progresses further the body starts retaining fluid. This condition is known as oedema and causes swelling of the ankles and, if fluid gathers around the lungs, shortness of breath with a general feeling of discomfort in the chest.

One of the most unpleasant features of this stage of renal failure is the inability to relax. The legs twitch as a feeling of unbearable tension builds up in the limbs. Mental concentration is reduced and sustained sleep becomes difficult. This is the case even though a patient can be feeling extremely tired and be spending a lot of time dozing in a fitful, fretful manner. Muscle cramps and tingling in the fingers and toes are also not unusual.

One of the only satisfying ways I found at that stage to be able to relax was to lie in a hot bath. I also felt a little better standing rather than sitting or lying down, but the feelings of general fatigue caused by the associated anaemia often made this far too exhausting except in short bursts. The twitching remains to some extent, even on dialysis. Patients who have transplants report how pleasant it is to be able to relax and sleep properly at night again. Not long ago one doctor suggested I took a valium-type drug to relieve the symptoms. This I refused, as I did not want to become drug-dependent.

As the kidneys get worse there is a constant demand from the doctors for blood samples. A kidney patient rolls up his or her sleeve almost by reflex action after a while. Some people hate having blood taken. Perhaps they have difficult blood vessels to find or perhaps it is a general dislike of needles. I never enjoyed looking at the blood being drawn out into the syringe and usually looked away while it was being done. As an outpatient often the worst thing is the wait. Even today too many hospitals have no coherent appointments system and patients have to sit around on hard chairs looking at out-of-date magazines in mind-numbing boredom anticipating the brief prick in the arm which is all they came to the hospital to have done.

As the moment of the first dialysis approaches urine tests are also important. The total output is measured and contrasted with the fluid input so that an idea as to how much fluid is being retained can be gained. Also the urine may for a while have been frothy and tended to resemble mild ale.

Treatment, short of the stage when dialysis is the only option, normally consists of a strict diet and drugs to control blood-pressure.

The most common cause of chronic kidney failure in Britain is glomerulonephritis. This is a term which covers an assortment of conditions involving lesions and inflammation of the glomeruli. Of the four to five thousand new kidney patients every year who reach end-stage renal failure about a third have one form or another of glomerulonephritis.

The cause of the condition is not known exactly but it is, in most cases, associated with the body's immune system. It is almost as if the body mistakes the glomeruli for some alien matter and starts to attack it.

Chronic renal failure can also be caused by a similar disease of other parts of the kidney, and not just the glomeruli.

Of the hereditary conditions polycystic is the most common. To have this or any other disease associated with genetic causes presents patient's families with a number of anxieties. One case of polycystic kidney disease in the family suggests another might occur. Young adults in such a family may worry about starting a family in case the trait is passed on to their children. Yet it is worth remembering that as inconvenient and uncomfortable as kidney failure can be it does not preclude a patient from living a very full life.

Whichever of the many forms of kidney disease a patient contracts, it is always a good idea to get it fully explained by the consultant. Just to be given a long medical name for an illness is not very satisfactory. I would suggest cross-questioning the consultant on the implications of the particular diagnosis. How will the type of illness affect the type of treatment? What is the usual prognosis and are any specific complications associated with this type of kidney failure? How long before end-stage renal failure is reached? Will the specific type of renal failure alter my chances of a transplant? Will some kidney function remain once dialysis has started? What research is currently underway relevant to my case?

Even if knowing the exact nature of one's kidney failure has no implications as far as treatment is concerned it is all part of feeling in control of the situation. I found it particularly useful to know about my particular form of renal failure in order to have a cómplete and well-rounded understanding of what was happening to me and what was likely to be done to me.

A doctor who will not explain to a patient precisely what is happening is, to my mind, not a good doctor. Medical secrecy often masks medical embarrassment or medical ignorance. From the doctor's point of view, it is a good investment of time to explain, even if he or she is very busy. It can save a lot of time later. A patient who knows what is happening is less likely to bother the doctor with trivial worries later on and is indeed more likely to stay well and need less medical attention in the future. Kidney patients find themselves serving a long-term sentence and can even become as knowledgable of their illness and treatment as many of the doctors who see them, particularly if the doctor is new to the speciality or the unit.

I have been very fortunate in having a consultant who is prepared to explain and discuss. Also at the minimal-care unit I see a doctor who is now used to my constant questioning and debating and who has learned over the years that I like to take, or feel that I am taking, decisions for myself.

Admittedly some people do not want to know the ins and outs of their medical condition. They are content to be told what pills to take and when and follow a simple dietary code. In such cases doctors may not volunteer much information, but if asked questions they ought to reply honestly and as fully as a patient wants. There is a tendency in some medical circles to underestimate the intelligence of patients and assume they cannot manage to digest information if it is in any way complicated. They too easily forget that people handle all kinds of complex information in their own lives and are perfectly able to understand medical matters as long as the explanation given is free from medical jargon.

How much a patient is told is, I would suggest, up to the patient. Some patients are quite happy to abdicate responsibility for themselves and hand all decisions over to the experts. They are happy to be compliant and obedient, though some doctors notice that these are the patients who release their grip on life with the least struggle.

I have heard doctors complain that, however careful they are to explain, patients invariably get hold of the wrong end of the stick and leave the surgery with some strange ideas about what is wrong with them and what is to be done. This I would suggest has nothing to do with the intelligence of patients but relates instead to doctors' communications skills.

A patient who has just been given some bad news about his or her health is not going to be very receptive to a detailed medical explanation. A doctor who uses long words, or who mumbles into notes, or is generally bored with having to explain things and answer questions is not going to communicate well. Patients can often be too ready to say they understand when they have not taken all the information in. They are too embarrassed about appearing slow on the uptake or about taking up too much of the doctor's time. Medical communication, I would suggest, also involves the doctor checking with the patient that he or she has understood, perhaps by asking them to explain things back. As long as the interview appears to be unhurried and the setting is not too formal I see no reason why medical information cannot be imparted successfully.

11
EATING AND DRINKING

Some people find the hardest thing to do when on haemodialysis is to keep to the fluid allowance. As the output of urine is reduced by kidney failure, and indeed falls to nothing if the kidneys are removed, it is not possible to drink normal quantities of fluid. A few pints down at the pub in the evening is not on; neither is it possible to keep drinking tea and coffee all day.

The amount a patient can safely drink is determined by the quantity of urine which can still be passed. The purpose of the fluid restriction is to prevent fluid accumulating in the body between dialysis sessions. The amount of fluid retained can be worked out simply by weight.

I normally hope to finish a six-hour stint of dialysis weighing 72 kilograms and expect to have increased my weight by between 1 and 2 kilograms when the time comes three or four days later to dialyse again. My ideal percentage weight increase between dialysis is thus 2 per cent.

If I accumulate too much fluid I experience a discomfort in the chest as the fluid tends to gather around the heart and lungs. Some people find their ankles swell. I have heard some stories of patients putting on 4 or 5 kilograms of fluid every time. One man I knew put on 7.5 kilograms of fluid in one week. Admittedly he was a big person and his percentage weight increase was 8 per cent. A smaller person putting on 4 kilograms can be increasing body weight by up to 10 per cent in four days and this can be dangerous.

To prevent myself from suffering the symptoms of being 'overloaded' I need to restrict my intake of fluid to 750 millilitres every day. I do not need to measure every cup of tea or glass of squash as, like most experienced dialysis patients, I can gauge quantities pretty accurately by eye and keep in my head a running tally of fluid intake. I have a cup which contains 150 millilitres which I use at breakfast. If I feel I do not need to drink all the tea I throw some of it away. There is no point in drinking it unless one is going to derive some enjoyment. Most mornings I find I start the day with 100 millilitres and I throw the rest of the tea away.

Mid-morning I might have a chance to have another cup of tea. Unless I am gasping I say no. There is no point in drinking just to be sociable. No one, I find, ever takes offence if an offer of a tea or coffee is politely refused.

With lunch I invariably have 150 millilitres of cold water. I need some liquid to down my alucap capsule and by that time of day I am normally in need of a little liquid refreshment. Unless I have eaten something salty I do not often feel thirsty. As I do not expel much liquid I do not get dehydrated. (In very hot weather, however, if I am perspiring a lot, I normally increase my fluid intake by up to 50 per cent and if I find by doing so that I am retaining too much fluid I reduce the intake accordingly.)

I sometimes have a small drink in the afternoon—tea or water—but always aim to reach 6 p.m. with my fluid tally no higher than 450 millilitres. This enables me to spend the evening with a proper drink. A glass tumbler holds around 300 millilitres and if the drink it contains also includes ice cubes it is quite easy to make it last and one can risk from time to time topping it up with extra ice. It is easy to work out roughly how much fluid an ice cube contains. Measure its width, length and height in centimetres, multiply the three figures together and the resulting number is its volume in millilitres. An ice cube 2 centimetres×2 centimetres×1 centimetre contains as little as 4 millilitres of liquid and yet can be as thirst quenching as 200 millilitres of ordinary drink.

As far as alcohol is concerned, there is little sense in drinking beer or cider. A pint is almost a day's allowance. A glass of wine is normally between 150 and 200 millilitres, but red wine is too high in potassium to be advisable and white wine, for the same reason, can only be consumed in moderation. I find an occasional glass of whisky a pleasant treat, especially if it is 'on the rocks'. The ice helps it last and whisky should only ever be sipped slowly. To be really self-indulgent a good single malt is preferable to a cheap blend.

A few practical points worth remembering: a can of drink always has its volume printed on the side. The average size for a can is 330 millilitres. A small bitter lemon or soda water contains 150 millilitres. The average disposable beaker contains just under 200 millilitres. I find it very useful to drink from the same cup and glass at home as I have measured them both and know exactly how much liquid each can hold. If you get a new drinks container it is a good idea to fill it full of water then pour the water into a measuring jug to check its exact capacity. Unless you are familiar with a particular mug or cup volumes can be misleading.

One of my gripes at the moment concerns fast food shops. Should I need a drink when I am out and about and go into a fast food establishment, pehaps on a railway station, their cold drinks are only available in beakers which contain at least 500 millilitres. To ask for a small drink is nigh on impossible. The only way to get one is to be prepared to pay the full price. I am told the tills are computerized and the staff have no discretion.

Sometimes when this happens I just ask for ice cubes and the staff are so surprised they give them to me free.

The moment of truth is the day of dialysis. Just before setting up the machine I stand on the scales and get the good or the bad news. Often I am surprised. I might think I have exceeded my fluid allowance by a little but the scales tell me otherwise. On other occasions I feel particularly virtuous and the scales give me a shock, and I find I have put on 2 kilograms. What can sway the calculation is the fact that many foods contain fluid. Ice cream, gravy and sauces boost the intake.

In practice I do not include these hidden quantities of fluid in my daily tally, but assume that if I keep my drink down to the ideal amount, the extras will not make an enormous difference. If, however, I wander over my fluid allowance by even as little as a cup of tea a day, that is an additional 0.6 kilograms added over four days which can push my weight up from an acceptable 1.5 kilograms increase to an increase over 2 kilograms and that extra weight can be felt.

Everybody on haemodialysis will develop, over time, their own method of restricting their fluid intake. I find setting targets during the day is a method that works for me. Others will find other methods. What I have noticed however are two things: those who keep their weight fluctuations to a minimum are those who keep in the best health on dialysis; they also do not have to suffer the discomfort of 'ultra-filtration' before dialysing each time. Ultra-filtration is the procedure whereby the patient is hooked up to the kidney machine so that excess fluid can be drained off before dialysis proper can start. It is time consuming and adds to the boredom of dialysis day by a significant margin.

Perhaps my most important discovery is that the busier one keeps in mind and body the less likely one is to yearn for the days of unrestricted fluid when cups of tea could be taken ad lib and a cold pint of lager was the perfect complement to a hot summer's day. There is however one compensation: it is very seldom that a haemodialysis patient has to get up in the night and trek to a cold bathroom for a pee.

Put any group of dialysis patients together in a room and the conversation quickly gets round to the same topic: food. Even add a few transplant patients and they will soon join in the conversation with gusto, though usually with such comments as, 'I remember the first time I had a bar of chocolate after my operation' or 'What I really enjoy now is bacon and eggs for breakfast with sausage, mushrooms, sauté potatoes and fried tomato!'

Keeping to the right diet is essential to good health on dialysis. Every patient is given a potassium, protein and salt allowance limit and some may also need to keep a close eye on phosphates.

While patients are often expected to be able to perform tasks as complicated as setting up and operating their own kidney machines at home, there is a tendency for too many renal nurses and dieticians to give oversimplified advice on food. This is an observation I have had endorsed by patients from many different units around the country who rather resent being patronized by being given lists of good foods and bad foods and little detailed information.

Renal patients are given the impression by dieticians that the culinary world is divided into foods which are goodies and others which are baddies. The reality, however, is that the amount of potassium consumed is as much determined by quantity consumed as by the mineral content of the food. By eating a lot of a food on the good list one can consume more potassium than by eating some of a food on the bad list in moderation. But patients are seldom given the detailed information required to make such judgments for themselves.

Chocolate, for instance, is almost universally banned by dieticians. Patients avoid even a single square like the plague. Yet a single square contains less potassium than a helping of

EATING AND DRINKING

boiled carrots, a food which is allowed.

Patients also need to know their blood results. Most units test blood samples for potassium and all the other indicators once a month. Having this information, and understanding it, is very useful when it comes to controlling one's own diet. It is of no help whatsoever for a doctor or renal nurse to interpret the results for the patient and then tick them off for being a 'naughty boy'. In almost any circumstances, medical staff talking of patients 'behaving themselves' or 'being naughty' is insulting to the patient and demeaning to the staff, and yet I have heard such expressions used and heard reports from other patients which suggest that such attitudes are still prevalent.

Dieticians often argue that many people cannot be trusted to monitor their own diets. The reason, I would contend, is that insufficient information is given to them. Patients, it is said, tend to cheat like naughty children, but it could well be said that if patients are treated as children they may behave as children. I believe that people given responsibility will rise to that responsibility and become more able to take control of their own lives. Some patients might prefer to be given a simple set of rules, a list of do's and don'ts; many others want facts. A valuable guide to renal diet, which gives much more information than ever I was given, is the one produced by the European Dialysis and Transplant Nurses Association called *Nutrition for Patients with Renal Failure*, edited by Marianne Vennegoor, the dietician at St Thomas's Hospital in London. She has also produced a cookbook for renal patients called *Enjoying Food on a Renal Diet*[1].

But the guide, *Nutrition for Patients with Renal Failure*, as excellent as it is, does not go far enough. For hard data I had also to go back to the statistical source: McCance and Widdowson's *The Composition of Foods*[2].

That enabled me to list all main foods and give their sodium, protein and potassium contents as related to a constant unit of weight, 100 grams (g). The full list is given in the

Appendix. This is how it works.

The potassium and sodium figures are all in millimoles (mmol), the standard measurement. A good rule of thumb is that a patient can safely consume up to 1 mmol of potassium for every kilogram of body weight. Thus my daily potassium limit should never go over 72 mmol and it is best to keep it a bit below. Almost everything contains some potassium. All food and drink must therefore be included in the daily calculation. Sodium too is expressed in terms of mmol and every patient will be set a limit or given a 'no added salt' diet and the advice to avoid salty foods. This will vary according to a number of factors, notably propensity to high blood pressure as salt causes blood pressure to rise.

Protein is expressed in terms of grams. Roast shoulder of lamb, for instance, contains almost 20 grams of protein per 100 grams consumed. Again, one's consultant will give a recommended figure of protein to be consumed in a day. By knowing the protein content of a food and the amount of that food one eats, it is possible to keep a daily running tally of protein intake. If I have 75 grams of roast shoulder of lamb for lunch, a modest helping, I will use up 15 grams of my daily allowance of 80 grams. The rule of thumb is that a haemodialysis patient needs between 1 and 1.2 grams of protein for every kilogram of weight. A person on a very restricted protein diet may be on an intake of as low as 0.6 grams per kilogram of weight.

It is also very important to remember that cooking and soaking affect the chemical content of certain foods. Identical weights of dried, raw and canned apricots have a potassium content which is totally different. The potassium contained in dried fruit is seven times greater than that in the same weight of fresh fruit.

People who are interested in working out their diet from first principles can use the charts *in* the Appendix to check the actual content of the foods they would like to eat. If the total of any one substance is too high, they can see which foods they can omit to get the level down.

[1]Published by King Edward's Hospital Fund for London, 2 St Andrews Place, London NW1 4LB.

[2]Fourth revised and extended edition, published by HMSO, London.

12

A WAY FORWARD

Temperamentally I was not designed for the twentieth century, I am suspicious of computers and all things 'high-tech' and, although I use a motor vehicle, I do not love it. Nevertheless, I do reflect on my good fortune in being born to live in the second half of this century, from the medical point of view.

Had I been born even thirty years earlier I would have died before reaching my fortieth birthday. So my gratitude goes out to the many hundreds of pioneers in the field of renal medicine whom I have never met and am never likely to meet, whose work contributed to my survival. I am sure many hundreds of other renal patients join me in saying that.

I am not here just thinking of the consultants and the scientists to whom the breakthroughs in treatment and technology have been attributed but of all the back-up staff involved: the laboratory cleaner, the porter who carried research material up to the professor's office, and the patients who allowed themselves to be used as guinea pigs so that new techniques could be tested. So many things, even the trivial things, that we do here on this earth affect others. Sometimes whole generations can be affected by one person and one deed. I and hundreds of other kidney patients are now alive because of the conscientious work of many thousands of people.

My gratitude also goes out to the many dozens of people in the medical world whom I have known and who have been involved in my treatment. Without their accumulated knowledge and effort I would not be where I am today. My gratitude is no less because I prefer to be a militant rather than a compliant patient. I see the medical staff as friends and fellow human beings and not as infallible supermen and women. Because I happen to have an expertise in the field of broadcasting that does not mean I am not also a collection of ordinary human faults. The same is true with medical staff: they have specialized training and a field of expertise, and yet at the same time exhibit all the symptoms of weakness which is the human lot.

The medical profession needs more than just its medical technology to treat patients. In the old days it was assumed that it needed to create an image of authority and infallibility to compensate for its areas of technical ignorance. While that attitude has modified considerably, there are still relics of it to be found. The hospital ward system itself is one such relic with its hierarchies and its rules.

The ward round is an extraordinarily inefficient way for consultants to find out how their patients are really doing. Patients still have to wait hours lying on a hospital bed before being granted a brief visit by the chief and his accompanying acolytes. They then have no privacy and no time to explain real worries and concerns. Ward bed curtains are not soundproof and there is no reason why a side room in the ward cannot be put aside as a consulting room to be visited by all mobile patients. I have seen patients fail to convey to their doctor what is really troubling them because of the intimidatory nature of the system.

Even in renal medicine, where technological intervention is of proven worth, more time needs to be spent by doctors in practising old-fashioned healing. Touch, time and talking are three valuable ingredients of healing now much neglected. There is one notable doctor in the renal unit at Canterbury who has not lost the art of touch and as a result he is extremely popular and well respected. My consultant Michael Goggin gives time to talk to patients and listen, and that is a strength which enhances his technical and scientific expertise.

The feed-back I have had from many patients, however, seems to suggest that too many doctors and nurses still prefer to keep their distance from their patients and hope that the authority which they claim, bolstered by the hospital system and the many petty rules they invoke, will cover up for their areas of medical uncertainty.

Some doctors must have a very odd view of the world. The world of hospital medicine is very enclosed. Doctors' friends tend to be other doctors. Doctors tend to marry doctors or nurses and their children often go into the medical professions. People from the outside world whom they do see tend to be identified by their diseases. One patient I know reports a stay in a ward of a leading teaching hospital. The consultant stood in the entrance to the ward with his entourage and said, 'Let me show you a polycystic kidney in bed one, a fistula in bed two and a recent transplant in number three . . . ' and so on round the ward, announcing every patient in a loud voice by his or her illness.

Nurses can equally well demean their patients by going too far in the other direction. I remember the case of one patient, let us call her Miss Emily Williams, a retired schoolteacher. The very fact that she was ill and exposed to public gaze in a ward had stripped her of much of her dignity. But whenever nurses, often very young students, spoke to her they addressed her in condescending tones as 'Emily'. 'Emily, it's time for a cup of tea,' 'Wake up Emily, it's time for your sleeping pill,' and so on. Miss Emily Williams was a person who in private life would have always been addressed as Miss Williams. She came from the class and generation when over-familiarity was not encouraged. The ward system had no way of maintaining the dignity and individuality so important to her well-being.

A vital element of maintaining dignity, individuality and thus hope, is to feel one has a degree of control over one's destiny. That is why I am such a strong advocate of patients' knowing what is happening to them and being involved in decisions. It is in no way a criticism of the medical profession. It is, to my mind, a vital complement to the expertise they have to offer. When one is very ill one is glad to be taken over by the staff to be helped through the crisis. But once, as is the case with kidney patients, the long-term treatment starts, patients should regain the reins of control as soon as possible. Serious illness saps one of confidence in life. One realizes one's mortality. Recovery is not so much regaining full health, that often never happens, as regaining one's confidence in self and the world around.

At a time of crisis those with faith find comfort in allowing God to take control. A friend of mine recently died from cancer. He was a man of great faith and during our last conversation he described to me how he prayed using the words of Christ just before his trial and crucifixion. 'O Lord, if it is possible let this cup pass from me, but not as I will but as thou wilt.'

A kidney patient, however, is not presented with the stark choices of a patient suffering from a terminal illness like cancer. He or she has hope. And once God has carried that person through the crisis he then obliges each of us to make the most of the life that is left. Each one of us has talents; surely it is our duty to make the most of them.

My work is as a journalist. Within the restrictions of my dialysis and diet I must make the most of the talents I have for writing and broadcasting and not allow the experience I have accumulated to go to waste. Other patients have other jobs, professions and callings. I am sure the best way any kidney patient can express his or her gratitude for treatment and survival is to return to normal productive life whenever and wherever possible.

I have found this approach valuable when I have been struck by doubt and conscience. Why, I sometimes ask, should I be worth to society the huge sums of taxpayers' money needed to keep me alive? It is an easy question to answer on behalf of someone else. I can say to a fellow kidney patient, if you are of infinite value in the sight of God, then you must be worth £15,000 a year of government money. But I cannot say that for myself. I feel I have to justify myself to society. In simple financial terms, the fact that I am earning and paying taxes and providing for my family lessens the debt.

Many people at the end of their life feel a sense of completion, of mission accomplished. As yet I feel I have much to do. I am sure this feeling is shared by many of my age and younger, and again that is an incentive to take control of an illness and not allow it to dominate beyond the initial periods of crisis.

But what would my approach have been if I had been struck by kidney failure much later in life? When I was on East Ward at the time my dialysis started there was a fellow patient who was blind and very deaf. He was kept alive for months by the best technical treatment and dedicated nursing. But towards the end more than one nurse I spoke to wondered if it was all worth it. He himself had said he now wanted to die and did not want any more treatment.

There comes a point in the treatment of cancer when curative treatment turns to palliative treatment. Exactly what happened to the patient I knew, I do not know. I know that he died after many months on the ward. Did he die despite all the medical intervention, or was it decided in the end to let him have his wish? There is a whole world of difference between euthanasia, the deliberate killing of a patient, and allowing someone to die of natural causes, giving treatment only to suppress the symptoms and distress associated with the illness near to death.

A WAY FORWARD

There is another area where doctors face difficult ethical choices. What should they do about the patient who refuses to take responsibility for him or herself, or who seems incapable of it. In the field of renal medicine this often means the patient who regularly fails to keep to the diet and fluid restrictions and omits to take medication prescribed. If the patient's health consistently reaches crisis point and the patient needs to be admitted and readmitted to hospital for emergency treatment, is there a point at which the doctor is entitled to say, 'Your refusal to do what is required of you is putting a strain on resources, denying other patients treatment, and in future I will not treat you'?

Many doctors might think of saying that, but few in practice ever would. They would continue to treat the patient, doing their best to suppress their irritation and anger, knowing that in the long term the patient is bound to die before emergency treatment can be administered.

I would suggest the patient's motives are examined more closely. Assuming the person is not mentally incapable of retaining instructions, most patients who fail to take responsibility for themselves may, consciously or unconsciously, be trying to say something. The unemployed youngster who constantly exceeds the drink limit may be saying, 'I am bored with this life which is unfair to me and therefore I will drink, enjoy myself while I can, because I don't see much of a future.'

The older patient with the same problem may have a different reason; 'I am getting on in years, and have had a good life, I know I am going to die, so I might as well enjoy myself while I can.'

The common, underlying factor is the sense of hopelessness. That is what needs to be addressed. For the patient to be admonished for being 'naughty' or subjected to unpleasant emergency treatment is not the long-term solution. Finding a hope and purpose in life is what is perhaps required.

I did not want to be ill and I did not expect to be ill. My

kidney failure demanded of my family and myself considerable adjustments. We moved house, to a different part of the country, and it resulted in Helen starting a whole new career. Many things have worked out very well. My routine of dialysis is not unduly burdensome and I have continued with my work. I still suffer some of the symptoms of renal failure, the twitching of the limbs in particular, but this has lessened over the months. As a result I have learned many things, especially about the medical profession. I hope, too, that I have learned some things about myself.

If my experience can be of any value to a new patient approaching the world of renal medicine with trepidation, I gladly share it. Renal disease is not pleasant but it is possible to live with it. What is vital is to nurture and develop the right attitude. Once the initial shock of diagnosis and crisis of acute illness is passed, it is essential once again to take control of one's own life. Work in co-operation with the medical profession, with you and the medical staff as equals. Understand what is being done to you and what you have to do. If you stay in charge of the management of the illness, you will be pleasantly surprised just how much life still has to offer.

Appendix

FOOD CHARTS

The following charts show the protein, sodium and potassium content of a wide range of foods. I hope I have included all the main foods a patient might want to eat. In working out the potassium, protein and sodium contents it is important to know the quantities of any food being cooked and served. To begin with this involves a lot of weighing, but in time it is possible to gauge the weight of food by eye with a fair degree of accuracy. Any food not on the list should be approached with caution until a dietician is consulted and its chemical and protein content known. Flavourings and sauces should also only be used in moderation as many have a high sodium content, particularly if commercially manufactured.

Knowing the protein and chemical analysis of food and the weight of food eaten it is very easy to keep a running tally of potassium, sodium and protein consumed during the day and to adapt intake to keep within the limits advised by the consultant. This way it is possible to enjoy moderate quantities of higher potassium foods and not be restricted to foods dubbed good by the dietician. It is possible, for instance, to incorporate more fruit and even a little chocolate into a renal diet if one is prepared to give up potatoes at most meals. Having the information means one can experiment more and, provided the blood tests are watched with care, it is possible to have complete control over one's diet and a greater freedom to enjoy food than when one is just following over-simplified rules.

Grains, Flours and Starches	Protein (grams per 100g)	Sodium (mmol per 100g)	Potassium (mmol per 100g)	Grams per average portion
Arrowroot	0.4	0.2	0.46	
Barley (pearl, boiled)	2.7	trace	1	
Bemax	26.5	0.17	25.6	
Bran (wheat)	14	1.2	29.7	
Bread				
currant	6.4	6.9	6.4	
malt	8.3	12.2	9.7	
soda	8	17.8	6.9	
white	7.8	23	2.6	33
wholemeal and brown	8.8	23	5.6	
Breakfast cereals				
All-bran	15	72.6	27	
Cornflakes	8.6	50	2.5	30
Grapenuts	10.8	28.6	6.9	
Muesli	12.9	7.8	15.4	60
Puffed Wheat	14.2	0.2	10	30
Ready Brek	12.4	1	10	
Rice Krispies	5.9	48	4.1	30
Shredded Wheat	10.6	0.3	8.4	50
Special K	18	38	4.8	30
Sugar Puffs	5.9	0.4	4.1	30
Weetabix	11.4	15.6	10.8	35
Chapatis				
made with fat	8.1	5.6	4.1	
made without fat	7.3	5.2	3.8	
Cornflour	0.6	2.26	1.56	
Custard powder	0.6	14	1.56	
Flour				
100% wholemeal	13.2	trace	9.2	
brown, 85% wholemeal	13.2	trace	7.2	
white, as used for breadmaking	11.3	trace	3.3	
white, plain household	9.8	trace	3.5	
self-raising	9.3	15	4.3	
Oatmeal (raw)	12.4	1.4	9.5	

APPENDIX

Porridge	1.4	25	1.1	180
Pasta				
Macaroni (boiled)	4.3	0.34	1.7	
Spaghetti				
boiled	4.2	0.09	1.3	200
tinned, in sauce	1.7	21	3.3	
Rice	2.2	trace	1	180
Rye flour (100%)	8.2	trace	10.5	
Sago (raw)	0.2	0.13	0.12	
Semolina (raw)	10.7	0.5	4.3	
Soya (low fat)	45	trace	52	
Soyaflour (full fat)	36.8	trace	42	
Tapioca (raw)	0.4	0.17	0.5	

Biscuits, Cakes and Puddings

	Protein (grams per 100g)	Sodium (mmol per 100g)	Potassium (mmol per 100g)	Grams per average portion
Biscuits				
Chocolate (fully-coated)	5.7	6.9	5.9	
Cream crackers	9.5	26.5	3.1	7
Crispbread				
rye	9.4	9.6	12.8	8
wheat, starch reduced	45	26	5.4	8
Digestive				
plain	9.8	19	4.1	15
chocolate	6.8	19.6	5.38	17
Ginger nuts	5.6	14.3	5.6	10
Matzo	10.5	0.74	3.8	
Oatcakes	10	53.5	8.7	
Sandwich biscuits	5	9.5	3	
Semi-sweet	6.7	17.8	3.6	7
Short-sweet	6.2	15.6	2.8	
Shortbread	6.2	11.7	2.3	
Wafers (filled)	4.7	3	1.9	10
Water biscuits	10.8	20.4	3.6	15

Cakes

Fancy iced cakes	3.8	10.8	4.3	30
Fruit cake				
plain	5.1	10.9	10	75
rich	3.7	7.4	11	
rich and iced	4.1	5.2	9.2	
Gingerbread	6.1	9.1	12	60
Madeira cake	5.4	16.5	3	
Rock cakes	5.4	20.9	5.4	
Sponge cake				
with fat	6.4	15.2	2.1	55
without fat	10	3.6	3.1	
jam filled	4.2	18	3.6	

Buns and pastries*

Currant buns	7.4	4.3	4.6	35
Doughnuts	6	2.6	2.8	50
Eclairs	4.1	6.9	2.4	
Jam tarts	3.5	10	2.8	40
Mince pies	4.3	14.8	3.8	60
Pastry				
choux, cooked	8.5	16.8	2.8	
flaky, cooked	5.8	20.4	2.3	
shortcrust, cooked	6.9	20.9	2.5	
Scones	7.5	34.8	3.6	30
Scotch pancakes	6.7	17.4	8.2	

Puddings

Apple crumble	1.8	2.9	2.6	
Bread and butter pudding	6.1	6.5	5.1	
Cheesecake	4.2	11.3	3	150
Christmas pudding	5.2	10.4	10	
Custard				
egg	5.8	3.4	4.4	
made with powder	3.8	3.3	4.3	
Custard tart	5.9	10.9	3.3	
Fruit pie				
with pastry top and bottom	4.3	9.1	3.1	
with pastry top	2	4.8	4.3	
Ice cream				
dairy	3.7	3.5	4.6	120–150
non-dairy	3.3	3	3.8	

APPENDIX

Jelly				
made with water	1.4	0.3	0.2	
made with milk	2.8	1.2	1.7	
Lemon meringue pie	4.5	8.7	2.1	
Meringues	5.3	4.8	2.3	
Milk rice pudding	3.4	2.2	4.4	120
Pancakes	6.1	2.2	3.6	
Queen of puddings	4.8	6.5	2.8	
Sponge pudding (steamed)	5.9	13.5	2.3	150
*Suet pudding (steamed)	4.4	10.4	2.3	
Treacle tart	3.8	15.6	3.8	
Trifle	3.5	2.2	3.8	
Yorkshire pudding	6.8	26	4.1	30 (1 small)
Dumpling	2.9	17.4	1.1	

*Note: *This is a section where the hidden salt content is likely to cause more problems than the protein or potassium. Salt can be kept to a minimum when cooking at home.*

Dairy Products

	Protein (grams per 100g)	Sodium (mmol per 100g)	Potassium (mmol per 100g)	Grams per average portion
Milk				
fresh, whole, sterilized, longlife and skimmed	3.4	2.2	3.6	
condensed and sweetened	8.3	5.6	10	
condensed, skimmed and sweetened	9.9	7.8	12.8	
dried (powder)	26	19	32.6	
dried, skimmed (powder)	36	23.9	42	
evaporated and unsweetened	8.6	7.8	10	
goats'	3.3	1.7	4.6	

Butter				
salted	0.4	37.8	0.38	
unsalted	0.4	0.3	0.38	
Cream				
double	1.5	1.2	2.0	30
single	2.4	1.8	3.1	30
sterilized and canned	2.6	2.4	3.1	
whipping	1.9	1.5	2.5	
Cheese				
Camembert type	22.8	61	2.8	40
Cheddar	26	26.5	3	30
cottage	13.6	19.6	1.4	60
cream	3.1	13	4.1	
Danish blue	23	61.7	4.9	30
Edam	24	42.6	4.1	30
Parmesan	35	33	3.8	
processed	21.5	59	2.1	
spread	18	50.9	3.8	20
Stilton	26	50	4.1	30
Yoghurt, low fat, natural	5	3.3	6.1	125–150
(*similar content for flavoured and fruit yoghurts*)				
Eggs				
boiled	12.3	6.1	3.6	48
fried	14.1	9.6	4.6	50
poached	12.4	4.8	3.1	
omelette	10.6			60 (1 egg)
scrambled				65 (1 egg)
Egg and cheese dishes				
(*sodium values can be reduced by adding less salt, but beware of sodium if eating out*)				
Cauliflower cheese	5.7	10.86	6.4	
Cheese soufflé	11.5	18	3.8	
Macaroni cheese	7.4	12	3.1	
Pizza (with cheese and tomato)	9.4	14.8	4.6	200
Quiche Lorraine	14.7	26.5	4.9	
Scotch egg	11.6	20.1	3.8	
Welsh rarebit	15.7	45	3.3	

APPENDIX

Fats and oils (non-dairy)
Margarine
Mayonnaise
Oil, olive
Oil, sunflower
Salad cream

All fats and oils are very low in protein content and potassium. Some, however, like butter, margarine and low fat spreads have added salt and the sodium content can be as high as 38mmols per 100g weight.

Mayonnaise, as it contains egg, will have a slightly higher protein and potassium count than pure fat.

Meat

	Protein (grams per 100g)	Sodium (mmol per 100g)	Potassium (mmol per 100g)	Grams per average portion

BACON: The sodium content will depend on the amount of salt used in curing the bacon. The protein content will depend on the ratio of fat to lean meat, as will the potassium content. The more fat the less protein and potassium.

Gammon				
lean, boiled	29.4	48	6.4	
lean and fat, boiled	24.7	41.7	5.4	
rashers, lean and fat, grilled	29.5	93	12	
Streaky bacon (lean and fat, fried or grilled)	24	82	7.4	30

(*Figures for back and middle cuts are very similar.*)

BEEF: Unless the beef has been salted the sodium figure is low but protein and potassium levels must be watched.

Brisket (lean and fat, boiled)	27.6	3.2	5.1	
Rump steak (lean, fried or grilled)	29	2.4	10	120–250

Sirloin (lean and fat, roast)	23.6	2.3	7.7	90
Silverside (lean, boiled and salted)	32	43.4	5.9	
Stewing steak (lean and fat, cooked)	31	15.6	5.9	
Topside (lean only, roast)	29	2.1	9.5	90

LAMB: All figures given for 100 g weight including bone where relevant.

Breast (lean and fat, roast)	19	3.2	6.4	
Chops, loin (lean and fat, grilled)	18	2.4	6.4	100–160
Cutlets (lean and fat, grilled)	15	2	5.4	
Leg (lean and fat, roast)	26	2.8	7.9	90
Scrag and neck (stewed, lean and fat)	25.6	10.4	4.9	

(*The added sodium is due to the salt in the cooking*)

Shoulder (lean and fat, roast)	20	2.6	6.6

PORK

Belly (lean and fat, grilled)	21	4.1	7.9	
Chops (lean and fat, weighed with bone)	22	2.9	7.7	100–160
Leg (lean and fat, roast)	27	3.4	9	90

(*For lean meat only the potassium content rises to 10 mmols.*)

Veal (roast or fried)	31.5	4.3	11

APPENDIX

Poultry and Game (without bone)	Protein (grams per 100g)	Sodium (mmol per 100g)	Potassium (mmol per 100g)	Grams per average portion

Potassium and protein contents vary not only according to the fat content but also, in some cases, according to the colour of the meat.

	Protein	Sodium	Potassium	Grams
Chicken				
dark meat (boiled)	29	4.1	5.9	
dark meat (roast)	23	3.9	7.4	100
white meat (boiled)	30	3	9.5	
white meat (roast)	26.5	3.1	8.5	100
Duck (lean, fat and skin, roast)	19.6	3.3	5.4	
Goose (roast)	29.3	6.5	10.5	
Grouse (roast)	31	4.2	12	
Partridge (roast)	37	4.3	10.5	
Pheasant (roast)	32	4.3	10.5	
Pigeon (roast)	28	4.8	10.5	
Turkey				
dark meat (roast)	28	3	6.9	100
white meat (roast)	30	2	8.7	100
Hare (stewed)	30	1.7	5.4	
Rabbit (stewed)	27	1.4	5.4	
Venison (roast)	35	3.7	9.2	

Offal

	Protein (grams per 100g)	Sodium (mmol per 100g)	Potassium (mmol per 100g)	Grams per average portion
Kidney				
Lamb (fried)	25	11.7	8.7	60 (2)
Ox (stewed)	26	17.4	4.6	
Pig (stewed)	24	16	4.9	

Liver

Calf (fried)	27	7.4	10.5	
Chicken (fried)	21	10.4	7.4	
Lamb (fried)	23	8.2	7.7	90
Ox (stewed)	25	4.8	6.4	
Pig (stewed)	26	5.6	6.4	
Oxtail (Stewed with bone)	12	3.1	1.6	
Tongue (ox, boiled)	19	43	3.8	
Tripe (stewed)	15	3.2	2.6	

Meat Products

	Protein (grams per 100g)	Sodium (mmol per 100g)	Potassium (mmol per 100g)	Grams per average portion

This section carries a sodium warning. Only if products are home produced can the salt content be controlled.

Beefburgers (fried)	20	38	8.7	60 (1)
Black pudding (fried)	13	53	3.6	50
Brawn	12	32.6	2.2	
Corned beef	27	41	3.6	30—slice
Faggots	11	35.6	4.6	
Haggis (boiled)	11	30	4.3	
Ham	18	54	7.2	50
Ham and pork (chopped)	14	47.4	5.9	
Luncheon meat	12.6	46	3.6	
Meat paste	15	32	4.1	
Sausages				
beef (fried or grilled)	13	48	1.8	80
frankfurters	9.5	42.6	2.5	60 (2)
liver	13	37	4.3	
pork (fried or grilled)	13.5	43.5	5.1	80
salami	19	80	4.1	30
saveloy	10	39	4.1	80 (1)

APPENDIX

Meat and Pastry Products	Protein (grams per 100g)	Sodium (mmol per 100g)	Potassium (mmol per 100g)	Grams per average portion

If made at home with little if any salt these products are a good bet on the protein and potassium front. Figures below are for shop-bought items with normal amounts of salt.

Cornish pasty	8	26	4.9	170
Pork pie (individual)	10	31	3.8	140
Sausage roll	7.5	24	3.1	60
Steak and kidney pie (pastry top only)	15	30	6.1	

The more pastry there is in a pie, the lower the protein and potassium readings will be.

Cooked Meat Dishes	Protein (grams per 100g)	Sodium (mmol per 100g)	Potassium (mmol per 100g)	Grams per average portion
Beef steak pudding	11	15.6	4.6	
Beef stew	10	17	5	
Bolognese sauce	8	19	8	
Curried meat	10	21	5.4	
Hot pot	9	29	11	
Irish stew	5	16	9	
Moussaka	9	14	9	
Shepherd's pie	7.6	20	6	

All dishes which contain vegetables can have potassium reduced by boiling and/or soaking vegetables in advance and then when eating the dish avoiding the gravy. Sodium content can be adjusted when cooking at home by varying the salt in cooking.

Fish (without bones)	Protein (grams per 100g)	Sodium (mmol per 100g)	Potassium (mmol per 100g)	Grams per average portion
Bloater (grilled)	24	30	11.5	
Cod				
baked	21	15	9	
fried in batter	20	4.4	9.5	130
grilled	21	4	9.7	
poached	21	5	8.5	
steamed	19	4.3	9	
Dogfish (fried in batter)	17	12.6	8	
Haddock				
fried	21	8	9	130
smoked and steamed	23	49	7.4	
steamed	23	5	8	
Halibut (steamed)	24	4.8	8.7	
Herring				
fried	23	4.3	11	90
grilled	20	7.4	9.5	
Kipper (baked)	25	43	13	120
Lemon sole				
fried	16	6	6.4	
steamed	21	5.2	7.2	
Mackerel (fried)	21	6.5	11	90
Pilchards				
(canned in tomato sauce)	19	16	11	80
Plaice				
fried in batter	16	9.5	6	
fried in breadcrumbs	18	9.5	7.2	130
steamed	19	5.2	7.2	
Saithe/Coley (steamed)	23	4.2	9	
Salmon				
canned	20	25	7.7	60
smoked	25	51	11	
steamed	20	4.8	8.5	
Sardines				
canned in oil, fish only	24	28	11	80
canned in tomato sauce	18	30	10.5	

APPENDIX

Skate (fried in batter)	18	6	6	
Sprats (fried, weighed with bones)	22	5.2	9.2	
Trout				
brown (steamed)	23.5	3.8	9.5	
sea (steamed)	23.5	9	9.5	
Tuna (canned in oil)	23	18	7	60
Whitebait (fried)	20	10	2.8	
Whiting				
fried	18	8.7	8.2	
steamed	21	5.6	7.7	

Shellfish

	Protein (grams per 100g)	Sodium (mmol per 100g)	Potassium (mmol per 100g)	Grams per average portion
Cockles (boiled)	11	153	1.1	
Crab				
excluding shell (boiled)	20	16	7	
canned	18	24	2.5	
Lobster (weighed without shell, boiled)	22	14	6.6	
Mussels (weighed with shell, boiled)	5.2	2.7	0.7	
Oysters (weighed with shell, raw)	1.3	2.6	0.8	
Prawns				
boiled in shells	8	26.5	2.4	
peeled and boiled	22	69	6.6	30
Scallops (steamed)	23	12	12	
Scampi (fried)	12	16.5	10	
Shrimps				
boiled	24	167	10.2	
canned	21	43	2.6	30
Whelks (weighed with shell, boiled)	2.8	1.7	1.2	
Winkles (weighed with shell, boiled)	3	8.5	0.7	

LIVING WITH KIDNEY FAILURE

Fish products	Protein (grams per 100g)	Sodium (mmol per 100g)	Potassium (mmol per 100g)	Grams per average portion
Fish cakes (fried)	9	22	6.6	120 (2)

(Salt content can be reduced when making fish cakes at home.)

Fish fingers (fried)	13.5	15	6.6	50 (2)
Fish paste	15	26	7.7	
Fish pie	7	9	8	
Kedgeree	13	34	4	
Roe (cod, fried)	21	5.6	6.6	

Vegetables	Protein (grams per 100g)	Sodium (mmol per 100g)	Potassium (mmol per 100g)	Grams per average portion

These tend to have a higher salt content when served in restaurants.

Artichokes				
globe (boiled and weighed as served)	0.5	0.26	3.6	
Jerusalem (boiled)	1.6	0.1	11	
Asparagus (boiled and weighed as served)	1.7	0.04	3	
Aubergine (raw)	0.7	0.1	6	
Beans				
baked (canned in tomato sauce)	5	21	7.8	40
broad (boiled)	4	0.9	5.9	
butter (raw)	19	2.7	43	
butter (boiled)	7	0.7	10.2	
french (boiled)	0.8	0.1	2.6	
haricot (raw)	21	1.9	30	
haricot (boiled)	6.6	0.6	8	100
runner (boiled)	2	0.04	4	75
Beansprouts (canned)	1.6	3.5	0.9	
Beetroot (boiled)	1.8	2.8	9	200

APPENDIX

Broccoli tops (boiled)	3	0.3	5.6	
Brussel sprouts (boiled)	2.8	0.1	6	80
Cabbage				
red (raw)	1.7	1.4	7.8	
savoy (boiled)	1.3	0.3	3	100
spring (boiled)	1.1	0.5	2.8	
white (raw)	2	0.3	7	
winter (boiled)	1.7	0.2	4.1	
Carrots				
old (raw)	0.7	4	5.6	
old (boiled)	0.6	2.2	2.2	70
young (boiled)	0.9	1	6.2	
young (canned)	0.7	12	2.2	
Cauliflower (boiled)	1.6	0.2	4.6	120
Celeriac (boiled)	1.6	1.2	10.2	
Celery (raw)	0.9	6	7	60

(Sodium and potassium are reduced by more than half on boiling.)

Chicory (raw)	0.8	0.3	4.6	
Cucumber (raw)	0.6	0.6	3.6	40
Endive (raw)	1.8	0.4	9.7	
Laverbread	3.2	24	5.6	
Leeks (boiled)	1.8	0.3	7	80
Lentils (split, boiled)	7.6	0.5	5.4	

(Values for sodium and potassium increase by three times when lentils are raw.)

Lettuce	1	0.4	6	25
Marrow (boiled)	0.4	0.04	2.1	
Mushrooms (fried)	2.2	0.5	14.6	
Mustard and cress (raw)	1.6	0.8	8.7	
Onion				
raw	0.9	0.4	3.6	
boiled	0.6	0.3	2	
fried	1.8	0.9	7	
spring (raw)	0.9	0.5	6	
Parsley (raw)	5.2	1.4	28	
Parsnip (boiled)	1.3	1.3	7.4	
Peas				
dried (boiled)	6.9	0.5	7	75
fresh (boiled)	5	trace	4.3	75
frozen (boiled)	5.4	0.1	3.3	
garden (canned)	4.6	10	3.3	
processed (canned)	6.2	14	4.3	
split (boiled)	8.3	0.6	7	

LIVING WITH KIDNEY FAILURE

Peppers, green (raw)	0.9	0.1	5.4	

(*Potassium reduced slightly on boiling.*)

Potatoes

baked	2.6	0.3	17	150
chips	3.8	0.5	26	

(*Potassium content can be reduced by soaking chips before frying but remains high.*)

crisps	6.3	24	30	30

(*One packet of crisps contains approximately 10 mmols of potassium.*)

Instant (made up as mashed potato)	0.2	11	8.7	
new (boiled)	1.6	1.8	8.5	
new (canned)	1.2	11	5.9	
old (boiled)	1.4	0.1	8.5	
old (chips, frozen and fried)	2.2	1.5	14	
old (mashed)	1.5	1	7.7	
roast	2.8	0.4	19	120
Radishes	1	2.6	6	
Spinach (boiled)	5	5.2	12.6	
Spring greens (boiled)	1.7	0.4	3	
Swede (boiled)	0.9	0.6	2.6	80

There is a traditional Orkney dish called clapshot which is a mixture of boiled and mashed swede and boiled and mashed potato. Given the high potassium content of potato, this is a very good way of bulking out the potato without overloading the potassium. Clapshot needs pepper and butter to taste.

Sweetcorn

kernels, canned	2.9	13.5	5	60
on the cob (boiled)	4	0.04	7	

Tomatoes

canned	1.1	1.3	6.9	
fried	1	0.1	8.7	
raw	0.9	0.1	7.4	60
Turnip (boiled)	0.7	1.2	4.1	
Watercress (raw)	2.9	2.6	8	
Yam (boiled)	1.6	0.7	7.7	

APPENDIX

Fruit	Protein (grams per 100g)	Sodium (mmol per 100g)	Potassium (mmol per 100g)	Grams per average portion
Apple				
cooking (baked without sugar)	0.3	0.1	3.3	120
cooking (stewed with sugar)	0.3	0.1	2.4	120
eating (weighed with skin and core)	0.2	0.1	2.4	120
Apricots				
canned	0.5	trace	6.6	
dried (raw)	4.8	2.4	48	
dried (stewed with sugar)	1.7	0.9	17	120
fresh (raw)	0.6	trace	8.2	
stewed with sugar (weighed with stones)	0.4	trace	6	120
Avocado pears	4.2	0.1	10	75
Banana (raw, weighed without skin)	1.1	trace	8.9	100
Bilberries (raw)	0.6	trace	1.9	
Blackberries				
raw	1.3	0.2	5.4	
stewed with sugar	1	0.1	4.1	120
Cherries				
eating (raw)	0.6	0.1	7.2	
stewed without sugar (weighed with stones)	0.4	0.1	5.6	120
Cranberries (raw)	0.4	0.1	3.1	
Currants				
black (raw)	0.9	0.1	9.5	
black (stewed with sugar)	0.8	0.1	7.4	120
dried	1.7	0.9	18	
red (raw)	0.9	0.1	7.2	
red (stewed with sugar)	0.8	0.1	5.6	120
white (raw)	0.9	0.1	7.4	
white (stewed with sugar)	0.8	0.1	5.6	120

Damsons				
raw (weighed with stones)	0.4	0.1	6.7	
stewed (weighed with stones)	0.4	0.1	6.1	120
Dates (dried, with stones)	1.7	0.2	16.7	15 (2)
Figs				
dried (raw)	3.6	3.8	26	
dried (stewed with sugar)	1.9	2	13.6	120
green (raw)	1.3	0.1	6.9	
Fruit pie filling (canned)	0.3	1.3	2	
Fruit salad (canned)	0.3	0.1	3.1	120
Gooseberries				
raw	1.1	0.1	5.4 (4.4 when ripe)	
stewed with sugar	0.9	0.1	4.1	120
Grapes				
black (raw)	0.6	0.1	8.2	
white (raw)	0.6	0.1	6.4	60
Grapefruit				
raw (whole fruit weighed)	0.3	trace	2.8	100
canned	0.5	0.4	2	
Greengages				
raw	0.8	trace	8	
stewed with sugar (weighed with stones)	0.6	trace	6	120
Guavas (canned)	0.4	0.3	3.1	
Lemon juice	0.3	0.1	3.6	
Loganberries				
raw or stewed	1	0.1	6.4	
canned	0.6	trace	2.5	
Lychees (canned)	0.4	0.1	2	
Mandarin oranges (canned)	0.6	0.4	2.3	
Mangoes (raw)	0.5	0.3	4.9	
Melon				
Canteloupe (raw)	1	0.6	8.2	120
yellow honeydew	0.6	0.9	5.6	120
watermelon	0.4	0.2	3	
Mulberries	1.3	0.1	6.7	
Nectarines (raw, weighed with stones)	0.9	0.3	6.4	

APPENDIX

Olives (in brine, weighed with stones)	0.7	78	1.8	
Oranges (raw, weighed with peel and pips)	0.6	0.1	3.8	140
Orange juice	0.6	0.1	4.6	
Passion fruit (raw, without skin)	2.8	1.2	9	
Peach				
canned	0.4	trace	3.8	120
dried (raw)	3.4	0.2	28	
dried (stewed)	1.3	0.1	10.5	120
fresh (raw)	0.6	0.1	6.7	
Pear (raw, weighed with skin and core)	0.2	trace	2.4	

(*Similar results if pears are canned. If pears are stewed in sugar the potassium reading falls to 2 mmols*)

Pineapple				
canned	0.3	trace	2.4	120
fresh	0.5	0.1	6.4	
Plums				
stewed with sugar (weighed with stones)	0.4	0.1	3.6	120
Victoria, raw (weighed with stones)	0.5	0.1	4.6	
Prunes (stewed with sugar and weighed with stones)	1.1	0.2	9.7	120

(*The potassium figure for raw prunes is double*)

Raisins (dried)	1.1	2.3	22	
Raspberries (raw)	0.9	0.1	5.6	

(*Similar figures when stewed with sugar, but figure for potassium drops to 2.7 mmols for canned raspberries*)

Rhubarb (stewed with sugar)	0.5	0.1	9.2	
Strawberries				
canned	0.4	0.3	2.5	120
raw	0.6	0.1	4.1	100
Sultanas (dried)	1.1	2.3	22	
Tangerines (raw, weighed with skin and pips)	0.6	0.1	2.8	60

LIVING WITH KIDNEY FAILURE

NUTS
All nuts have dangerously high potassium levels. Some are also high in protein and salt. Potassium levels for almonds (22 mmols per 100 g), peanuts (17 mmols), coconut (11.3 mmols), chestnuts (12.8 mmols) are too high for any impulse nut eater with kidney failure even to attempt. Roasted peanuts are also high in salt and peanut butter too is very high in sodium, protein and especially potassium.

SUGAR
Pure white sugar is protein, sodium and potassium free and is therefore a good source of energy but bad for the teeth. Watch out however for demerera sugar (potassium 2.3 mmols) and treacle. The potassium level of golden syrup is 6.1 mmols per 100 g weight and black treacle has an astonishing potassium content of 37.8 mmols.

Preserves

	Protein (grams per 100g)	Sodium (mmol per 100g)	Potassium (mmol per 100g)	Grams per average portion
Cherries (glacé)	0.6	2.8	0.5	
Honey	0.4	0.5	1.3	15
Jam	0.5	0.5	2.6	15
Lemon curd (home made)	3.3	6.5	1.7	
Marmalade	0.1	0.8	1.1	15
Marzipan	8.7	0.5	10.2	
Mincemeat	0.6	3.6	4.9	

APPENDIX

Sweets	Protein (grams per 100g)	Sodium (mmol per 100g)	Potassium (mmol per 100g)	Grams per average portion
Boiled sweets	trace	1.1	0.2	
Chocolate				
milk	8.4	5.2	10.8	60
plain	4.7	0.5	7.7	
Bounty bar	4.8	7.8	8.2	58
fancy and filled	4.1	2.6	6.1	
Mars bar	5.3	6.5	6.4	68
Fruit gums	1	2.8	9.2	
Liquorice allsorts	3.9	3.3	5.6	
Pastilles	5.2	3.3	1	
Peppermints	0.5	0.4	0.2	
Toffee	2.1	14	5.4	

Drinks	Protein (grams per 100g)	Sodium (mmol per 100g)	Potassium (mmol per 100g)	Grams per average portion
Coca cola etc	trace	trace	trace	
Coffee				
brewed from ground and roasted beans	trace	trace	1.7	
instant (unmade-up powder)	trace	trace	102	
Horlicks		15	19	
(Ovaltine is also high in sodium and potassium)				
Pineapple juice (canned)	0.4	0.1	3.6	
Ribena (undiluted)	0.1	0.9	2.2	
Tea	trace	trace	0.4	
Tomato juice	trace	10	6.6	

SOUP

All canned and packet soups are high in sodium (up to 20 mmols per 100 g). Many, depending on ingredients, are also high in potassium (eg canned tomato soup potassium level is 4.9 mmols).

Protein, sodium and potassium levels of home made soup can be varied to requirements but soups quickly use up the fluid allowance and are not recommended to kidney patients.

Alcoholic Drinks

	Protein (grams per 100g)	Sodium (mmol per 100g)	Potassium (mmol per 100g)	Grams per average portion
Beer	0.3	1	1	

(Stout and strong beers have potassium levels of approximately 2 mmols per 100 ml.)

Cider	trace	0.3	2	
Fortified wines and liqueurs			1.5–3	

(The sweeter the drink, the higher the potassium level.)

Wine				
red			3.3	
rose			1.9	
sparkling, white			1.5	
white (dry)			1.6	
white (medium)			2.3	
white (sweet)			2.8	

Spirits are potassium, sodium and protein free.

© Crown copyright 1990/Reproduced with the permission of the Controller of Her Majesty's Stationery Office.